Strength Training for Seniors

Strength Training for Seniors

Michael Fekete, CSCS, ACE

KEY PORTER BOOKS

Library and Archives Canada Cataloguing in Publication

Fekete, Michael
   Strength training for seniors / Michael Fekete.

ISBN 1-55263-660-7

1. Exercise for older people. 2. Weight training. 3. Muscle strength.
4. Physical fitness for older people. I. Title.

RA781.F44 2005   613.7'0446   C2004-907065-7

The publisher gratefully acknowledges the support of the Canada Council for the Arts and the Ontario Arts Council for its publishing program. We acknowledge the support of the Government of Ontario through the Ontario Media Development Corporation's Ontario Book Initiative.

We acknowledge the financial support of the Government of Canada through the Book Publishing Industry Development Program (BPIDP) for our publishing activities.

Key Porter Books Limited
Six Adelaide Street East, Tenth Floor
Toronto, Ontario
Canada M5C 1H6

www.keyporter.com

Text design: Peter Maher
Electronic formatting: Jean Lightfoot Peters

Printed and bound in Canada

05 06 07 08 09 6 5 4 3 2 1

Contents

Foreword

This is a book about becoming stronger, and rewinding your biological clock for more energy, vitality, well-being, and enjoyment of life through strength training.

I have been training seniors successfully now for many years. I enjoy knowing that I am a positive force in the lives of others. To see the weak become strong, the sedentary active, and the disabled and dysfunctional capable and able is worth more than all the world titles I won as a master athlete.

From the very beginning of my career as a coach, strength and conditioning specialist, rehab specialist, and personal trainer, I was inspired by a statement I read some 30 years ago by Henry David Thoreau. It went something like this: "I know of no more encouraging fact than our unquestioned ability to elevate our own life and to promote positive changes in the lives of others by intelligent, persistent, and focused effort, by leaving nothing to chance."

I hope that this book will not only inspire seniors to train in a safe and effective way to gain more strength, but will also provide them with a practical, no-nonsense approach to fitness training in general.

In my studies and everyday aspirations as a trainer, I was guided and influenced by the work of two great Canadian scholars, Roy Sheppard and Kenneth Sidney, leading Canadians both and two of the world's best exercise scientists. Their books, studies, and articles not only provided insight into the various aspects of aging, but motivated me to apply that knowledge for the practical purpose of enabling seniors to become stronger and fitter.

As to the methodology of strength training, my thanks go to Dr. Tudor O. Bompa whose excellent books and courses at York University gave direction and cohesion to my ideas regarding strength training.

But the greatest professional inspiration, motivation, and encouragement came from my clients, who were able to put up with my unrelenting demands for commitment, discipline, persistence, and focus, as well as with my often unusual training methods while I myself was learning. Through learning and experience, we all became better at training. I was just as happy to see one who was sedentary and almost disabled get up from a chair and walk, as I was delighted to see another win master championships. To them I want to extend my thanks.

"Scientists have yet to discover the philosopher's stone that will confer immortality. However, the ability of regular exercise to reduce biological age by 10 to 20 years is no mean miracle. Indeed, I know of no other therapy that could achieve comparable results."
—*Roy J. Shephard*[1]

As one of the many results of social and scientific advancements, we live longer. During the last 50 years, our life expectancy has increased dramatically. The number of years ahead of us are constantly growing. In 1930 the total life span of the Canadian male and female averaged 60.0 and 62.1 years respectively. Due to advancements in health care, sanitation, nutrition, and a higher standard of living, by 1990 these figures had increased to 70.0 and 80.7 years respectively.[2]

These are impressive numbers even when we recognize that the full potential for longevity is far from being realized due to factors such as pollution, bad eating habits, insufficient exercise, and the increase in certain diseases. But seniors want more than statistical numbers showing a mere extension of life. They want enjoyment, independence, and an enhanced ability to carry on with the activities of daily living, such as caring for themselves. During the last couple of years they are venturing even further. They are actively seeking and gaining access to recreational and athletic activities that they could not explore before their retirement.[3] They want to live those extra years of life to the fullest, with vitality and energy.

While a decade ago a senior citizen was expected to slow down and take a rest, now the trend is to add more and more activities to the list. Wherever you go today, you can see seniors on trails, in canoes, on bicycles. They not only do things that they were not supposed to do a few decades ago, but they do it well. A good friend of mine who is 80 years old and several times a master champion told me a story. He was kayaking on Lake Erie last year, warming up for his training session. He said that as he got older, his old bones and muscles needed more and more gentle warming up before he was able to paddle hard for a few hours on rough water. A group of youngsters paddled by and he asked if they minded if he cruised with them. They said as a rule, they wouldn't mind; however, because they wanted to kayak to an island that was quite a distance away, they would prefer that he didn't. On top of it, they told him that they did not like to wait for slowpokes. Les arrived at that island a good thirty minutes ahead of them. He could not hold back a sarcastic remark when he saw them pulling their kayaks up the shore: "I had never thought of it before, but now I know how it feels to wait for slowpokes."

Physical activity for seniors is just as important, if not more so, than it is for other age groups. Older adults came to recognize that *the "fountain of youth" is movement.* Their desire to exercise is becoming stronger and stronger. Seniors as an age group tend to become physically more active than teenagers. The image of sedentary, physically inactive seniors is becoming a matter of the past. Now senior citizens, instead of slowing down and taking a rest, fully realize that they can't afford to slow down, so they halt many of the undesirable effects of aging by being physically active. Not only can they check the effects of aging, but they can reverse them.

Recently, Canada took a leading role in recognizing the significance of training older adults when the Canadian Centre for Activity and Aging, funded by a three-year grant from Health Canada, developed guidelines for training older adults and published a National Blueprint Document. Canada is also the moving force behind forming an international

1. R.J. Shephard, *Aging, Physical Activity and Health* (Champaign, Illinois: Human Kinetics, 1997), p. 29.

2. K.G. Kinsella, "Changes in Life Expectancy," *American Journal of Clinical Nutrition* 55 (1992): 1196S–1202S.

3. R. Krongold, unpublished lecture notes, 2003.

coalition to draft a document that recommends international training guidelines for training seniors. Accepted by the Sixth World Congress on Aging and Physical Activity, held August 3–7, 2004, in London, Ontario, and endorsed by the World Health Organization, these guidelines for safely and effectively training seniors will now be implemented all over the world, elevating the quality of life for millions.

There have been many books written on various forms of physical training for seniors. In Canada, we are especially fortunate to have some of the most recognized international experts on aging and physical activity. They are doing a terrific job in conducting important research, providing fitness professionals with valuable information, and promoting active lifestyles for older adults. These experts are also influencing our governmental and social agencies to invest more money, time, and effort in a national program of making physical activity an integral part of the lives of seniors. Today, more than ever before, we have an increased number of older adults walking; jogging; participating in flexibility, yoga, and pilates classes; and engaging in master events in every sport. This trend, for the good of all of us, is growing. Besides gardening, seniors do trail walking, play tennis, golf, kayak, and bike. There were more athletes participating in the World Master Games than in the Olympics, and I could go on at great length about the increase in adult participation in various physical activities.

Among all this momentum for a more active adult lifestyle, why is there a need for a book on strength training? Why is strength such an important aspect of our overall fitness?

Strength, as opposed to weakness, is the ability to defeat gravity and resistance and move with vitality and vigor. Strength, as opposed to giving way, succumbing, crumbling, and failing, is the energy that enables us to produce force, to perform skilled and powerful motions. *Strength provides the impulse, dynamics, and momentum behind the ability of the human body to act with force and energy.* Without sufficient strength, we would decline, give way, crumble, and fail. Without strength, we would not be able to do any of the activities that make us healthy and fit adults.

General fitness includes strength, endurance, flexibility, coordination, and balance. Among the various aspects of being physically able, *strength is the basic quality that provides the necessary foundation and influences our performance of all the other capacities that make up fitness.*

Strength has an overall effect on all other aspects of fitness. It has been established that half of the age-related decline in aerobic capacity is due to a loss of muscle mass.[4] Fortunately, strength can be improved upon safely and effectively until a very late age. It has been demonstrated that even 90-year-old seniors can participate and benefit from serious strength training.[5] Several studies prove that muscle strength can be improved by as much as 66 percent at a very late age.[6]

General fitness and its most important aspect, strength, decline as we age. One of the effects of this decline is the loss of lean muscle tissue, which means loss of strength. But this decline can be slowed down, stopped, and in many cases turned around and the quality of our life can be improved by exercise. Strength is the spring that makes our biological

4. S.L. Charette, L. McEvoy, G. Pyka, C. Snow-Harter, and G. Riffat, "Muscle Hypertrophy Response to Resistance Training in Older Women," *Journal of Applied Physiology* 70 (1991): 1912–1916.

5. E.N. Booth, S.H. Needen, and B.S. Tseng, "Effect of Aging on Human Skeletal Muscle and Motor Function," *Medicine and Science in Sports and Exercise* 26 (1994): 556–560.

6. T.L. Dupler and C. Cortes, "Effects of Whole Body Resistive Training in the Elderly," *Gerontology* 39 (1993): 314–319.

clock tick—fortunately, this spring can be rewound until a very late age for our clock to tick on vigorously. The seniors I train for strength, and the master athletes I know, not only slow down the process of muscle loss, but many of them stop it and reverse it. But the benefits of exercise are more extensive than that.

It is a proven fact that, as opposed to those who do not exercise regularly, physically active seniors can rewind their biological clock and enjoy the following benefits of exercise:

1. better health that includes:

    - improved cardiovascular function
    - improved pulmonary function
    - favorable changes in blood lipids
    - improved hormonal activities
    - improved enzymatic activities
    - healthier glucose levels
    - improved immune function and resistance to diseases such as cancer
    - better sleep
    - improved cognitive function
    - increased ability to cope with stress, reduced anxiety and depression, enhanced moods, and an improved ability to relax
    - more effective immune system
    - social benefits such as increased contacts, friendships, support groups, and involvement in sports events that in turn have positive effects on mental health

2. improved fitness that includes:

    - gain in strength
    - increased aerobic endurance
    - improved flexibility and range of motion
    - better coordinative and balancing skills
    - improved velocity of movements (increased muscle speed)
    - healthier body composition (higher lean muscle-to-fat ratio)
    - better posture and gait

I could go on at length about the list of benefits that elevate the quality of life of active adults. I could also talk endlessly about the various physical and mental/emotional improvements that exercise in general have made in the lives of my "mature" clients. But this book is about improving our strength through serious strength training, so I will deal with the specific benefits of this very important training modality.

Over the years as a personal trainer and strength and conditioning specialist, I have had the opportunity to see and experience the benefits of various exercise modalities, such as aerobic training, flexibility training, and strength training. While I wholeheartedly agree that it is important to balance aerobic, flexibility, and strength training according to the individual needs of each person, strength training is of paramount and primary importance for seniors because strength has such an important effect on the other aspects of fitness.

I actively train for endurance events that involve swimming, kayaking, biking, and running. At age 53, I won the masters category in one of the most gruelling, multisport events, the Extreme Quadrathlon, held in Courpiere, France. This race was a 10k swim, 40k kayak, 200k bike ride, 42k run—nonstop. One would think that for endurance events like that, 90 percent of my training should have been aerobic. However, in fact, it was strength training that was the most important aspect of my exercise regimen and I gained more benefits from strength training than from all other forms of exercise altogether. During the course of my professional career as a coach and trainer, I have applied every form of physical exercise to improve the fitness of my clients and the athletes I train. I have found that it is strength training that brings about the widest range of immediate, maintainable, and long-lasting physical and mental/emotional benefits. Recent research proves that even with the very elderly and the very weak, effective strength training increases independent function skills and produces significant improvements in stair climbing, getting up from the floor, rising from the chair, and walking speed.[7]

What are the physical benefits of strength training?

- stronger muscles, bones, tendons, and ligaments
- reducing the negative effects of osteoporosis
- improved function, coordination, skill, and balance
- improved range of motion
- better posture
- reduction in low back problems
- improved body composition by increasing lean muscle mass
- higher metabolic rate (muscle is the most metabolically active tissue that burns fat by its mere existence)
- improved protein synthesis
- improved cardiac function
- improved respiratory function through strengthening of chest muscles
- easing the pain of osteoarthritis and rheumatoid arthritis
- better glucose utilization
- faster gastrointestinal transit
- decrease in blood pressure
- improvement in blood lipids
- improved hormonal and local enzymatic activity
- more effective immune system
- improved physical appearance

If we compare the physical benefits of strength training to those of exercise in general, we cannot fail to notice that strength training alone includes almost every physical benefit of all other forms of exercise.

Of course, we are able to gain and enjoy the benefits of improved strength only if we practise strength training safely, effectively, and systematically, otherwise the gains are short-lived and we run the risk of injuries, burnouts, lack of progress, and, ultimately, failure.

7. J. Bean, S. Herman, D.K. Kieley, D. Callahan, K. Mizer, W.R. Frontera, and R.A. Fielding, "Weighted Stair Climbing in Mobility-Limited Older People: A Pilot Study," *Journal of American Geriatrics Society* 50 (2002): 663–670.

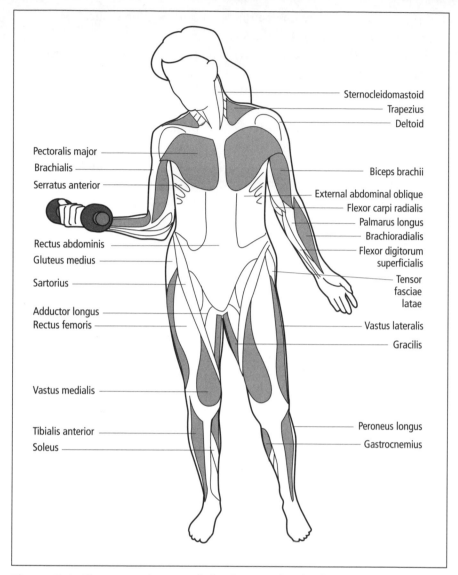

Figure 2.1: The musculature of the human body, front view.

Most seniors embark on a strength-training program without bothering to get acquainted with the source and origin of their strength: the *muscular system*. If we are familiar with the location and function of our muscles and have a basic knowledge of the anatomical, physiological, and biomechanical principles behind the functioning of our musculature, we will be more successful in improving our strength. In addition, we need to acquire a practical knowledge of the terminology used in strength training, in order to understand descriptions and follow instructions.

Every movement we make, and an overwhelming majority of our bodily functions, relies on the muscular system. Muscles work almost unnoticed with every heartbeat, with every breath we take, as we stand motionless, or when we sleep. In fact, there is not one moment when several muscles or muscle groups are not performing some work.

Besides the ability to perform work, muscles have another essential capacity: of all the tissues in our bodies, they are the best at responding and adapting to the specific demands imposed upon them and more—

Understanding the Basis of Our Strength

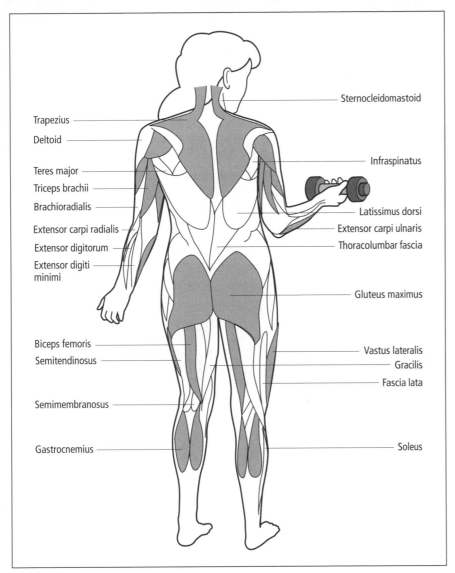

Trapezius
Deltoid
Teres major
Triceps brachii
Brachioradialis
Extensor carpi radialis
Extensor digitorum
Extensor digiti minimi
Biceps femoris
Semitendinosus
Semimembranosus
Gastrocnemius

Sternocleidomastoid
Infraspinatus
Latissimus dorsi
Extensor carpi ulnaris
Thoracolumbar fascia
Gluteus maximus
Vastus lateralis
Gracilis
Fascia lata
Soleus

Figure 2.2: The musculature of the human body, rear view.

they are able to maintain this ability longer and better than any other organ or bodily system. As a bonus, they also stimulate other organs, bones, tendons, ligaments, and our cardiovascular, metabolic, and immune systems to go along with and be part of this positive adaptation. *This extreme adaptability of the muscles and the stimuli they provide for the whole body makes strength training the most effective form of exercise for the elderly.*

For a long time, the aging process seemed to be associated with a steady and radical decrease in strength, power, and function. This process can be altered, however, with regular strength training.[1]

The muscles we are interested in when we talk about strength training are the *skeletal* muscles, which are attached to bones that serve as levers. The muscles attached to our bones produce a movement of body parts in relation to one another and/or the movement of our bodies against an outer force or resistance. Muscles create the tension necessary to hold us upright against gravity, to hold an object, or to maintain correct posture.

1. H. Akima, Y. Kano, Y. Enomoto, M. Isuzu, M. Okada, Y. Oishi, et al., "Muscle Function in 164 Men and Women Aged 20–84 Yr," *Medicine and Science in Sports and Exercise* 33 (2001): 220–226.

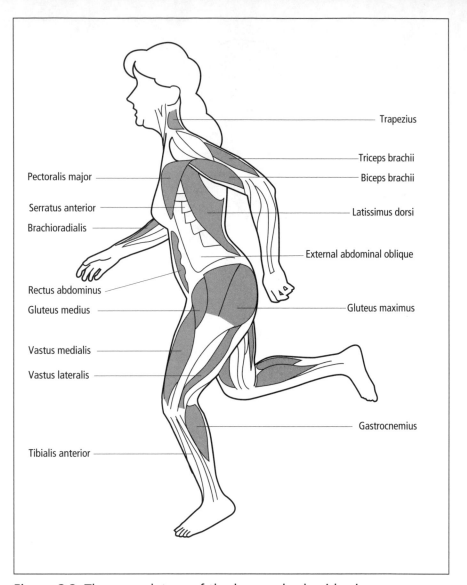

Figure 2.3: The musculature of the human body, side view.

Muscles are engines that are attached to our bones via cables that are called *tendons*. Skeletal muscles are the muscles of the arms, the torso, and the legs—generally speaking, the muscles that that we use to produce motion, locomotion, and to maintain a certain posture.

There are muscles that are not attached to bones, for example, the muscles of the heart and the muscles in the walls of the intestines. The primary function of these muscles is not to produce the motion of a certain body part in relation to another and/or to provide resistance against an outer force or to maintain a certain posture, but to help perform a bodily function.

Skeletal muscles have an amazing ability to relax, contract, and produce force that results in movement. Skeletal muscles respond to exercise or the lack of exercise faster and more efficiently than any other part or system of our bodies. Exercise that provides positive stimulus for the muscles will result in bigger and stronger muscles. Lack of exercise will lead to reduced and weaker muscles, and inappropriate exercise will

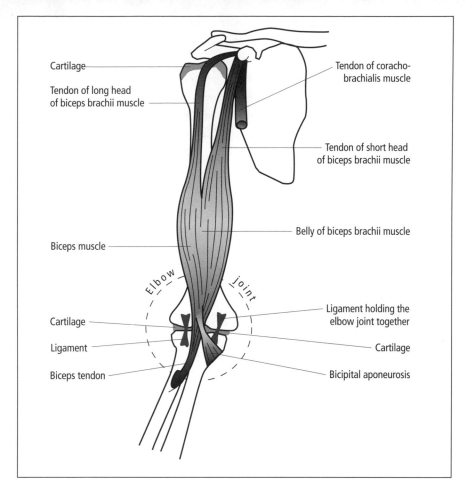

Figure 2.4: The muscles, tendons, bones, ligament, and joint.

cause injuries, wear and tear, and a gradual degradation of the muscular system.

The force created by our muscles is transferred to our bones via tendons. Tendons are a less active form of tissue and serve as cables between the force-producing muscle engine and the levers that are our bones. The motion produced usually happens around a *joint* or around several joints if we talk about complicated movements. Joints are usually located at the ends of our bones and are held together by *ligaments*. Our joints are lined and padded with *cartilage*, which acts as a lubricated shock absorber.

The fuel our muscles use is found and stored in different forms in the muscles, around organs, under the skin, in the blood, and in the liver. In whatever form and at whatever location this fuel is stored, it has to be broken down through various processes into adenosine triphosphate (ATP), which provides the direct energy for muscle action. The amount of fuel used for muscle action is measured in *calories*. Just as an engine produces exhaust fumes, the muscles using the fuel also produce various waste products that must be absorbed and processed, removed, and sometimes reused by a series of different metabolic processes.

Muscle tissue, unlike fatty tissue, bones, tendons, ligaments and the skin, is a *metabolically active tissue*. The bigger and more active our muscles are, the more calories they burn. They burn calories even when they are at rest. While we sleep, our skeletal muscles burn more than 25 percent of the calories we use.

As we know, our skeletal muscles are attached to our bones by tendons and they set the bones in motion with a series of coordinated contractions. Because muscle action exerts force on our tendons, bones, and the joints that are held together by ligaments, this stimulating force results in positive adaptations, not only in the muscles themselves but also in these tissues. This means that *through strength training, we get not only stronger and bigger muscles, but stronger and more robust bones, tendons, and ligaments as well.* The overall result is not only a greater capacity to perform work, but an increased protection against injuries.

Muscles are made of *fibers* and the number of fibers in a muscle is genetically determined. When we increase the size of our muscles, it is the result of extra proteins being built into the individual muscle fibers and not the result of an increase in the number of individual muscle fibers.

There are two primary muscle fibers: *slow-twitch* (Type I) and *fast-twitch* (Type II). When we perform cyclical-repetitive movements at a relatively low level of force for a long time, such as distance running, walking, or distance biking (forms of exercise we call "aerobic"), we rely mostly on the slow-twitch muscles to do the work. When we produce a high level of force for a shorter period—such as jumping, sprinting, or lifting a heavy weight (forms of exercise we call "anaerobic")—we rely mainly on the fast-twitch muscles. During regular strength training that consists of several *repetitions* performed in several *sets,* both muscle types participate equally in performing the movements.

A large pool of muscle fibers activated by the same motor nerve is called a *motor unit.* When a *nerve impulse* originating from the brain activates a motor unit, all fibers in that unit contract with maximal force. The overall force of the movement produced is regulated by the number of motor units participating in the movement.

Depending on the amount of force required to perform a particular movement against a certain resistance at a certain speed, the central nervous system selectively recruits a smaller or a larger number of motor units within the particular muscle or muscle group responsible for executing the movement.

For fine, coordinative, complicated movements (such as doing up the top button of a shirt) performed at a relatively low level of force, we use a large number of smaller motor units, found in the arms and the hands.

For crude and relatively simple movements performed at a relatively high level of force (such as jumping over a puddle), we use a smaller number of large motor units, such as the muscles in the legs and the trunk.

The major muscles participating in and providing most of the force needed for executing a certain movement or series of movements are called *prime movers.* Those providing assistance through stabilizing the posture required for the movement or helping direct the movement are called *secondary movers.*

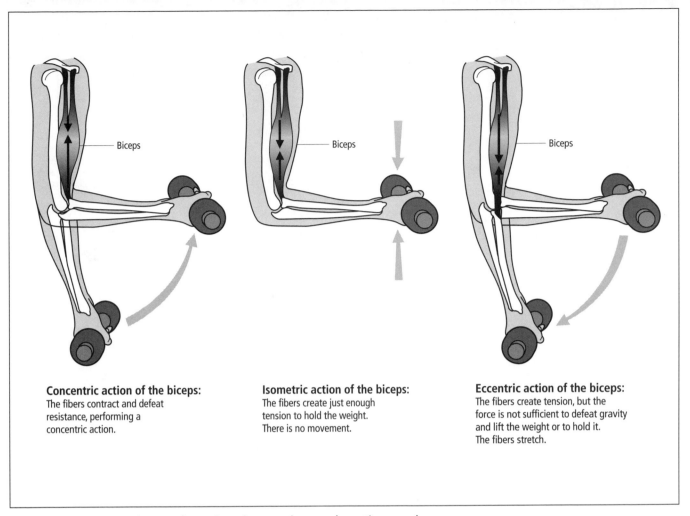

Concentric action of the biceps:
The fibers contract and defeat resistance, performing a concentric action.

Isometric action of the biceps:
The fibers create just enough tension to hold the weight. There is no movement.

Eccentric action of the biceps:
The fibers create tension, but the force is not sufficient to defeat gravity and lift the weight or to hold it. The fibers stretch.

Figure 2.5: Concentric muscle action, isometric muscle action, and eccentric muscle action.

Muscle actions that produce a force that defeats the resisting force as the muscle fibers shorten are the result of concentric or positive actions. All pushing, pulling, or lifting exercises where body parts move in relation to one another and successfully overcome resistance are the result of *concentric* or *positive* actions.

Muscle actions that produce a force equal to the resistive force or to the force of gravity but produce no movement are called *isometric* actions. All "holding" actions in which body parts do not move in relation to one another and the muscle participating in the action neither shortens nor lengthens but maintains a certain tension are called isometric actions.

Muscle actions in which the force produced is weaker than the resistive force or gravity and the activated muscle is forced to lengthen are called *eccentric* or *negative* actions. The fundamental movements resulting from the contraction (shortening) of muscles are: *flexion, extension, abduction, adduction,* and *rotation.* There are many other motions and combinations of motions. To understand the *biomechanics* of movements, it will suffice to get acquainted with these five basic motions.

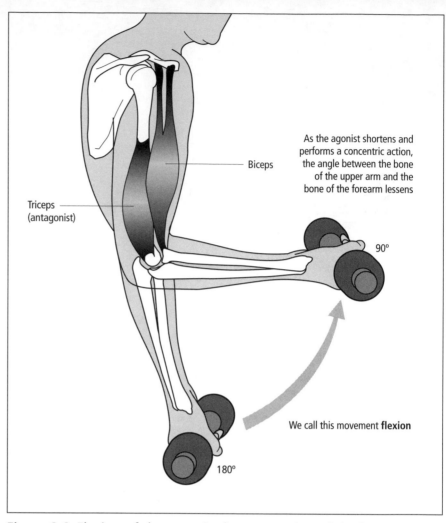

Biceps

Triceps
(antagonist)

As the agonist shortens and
performs a concentric action,
the angle between the bone
of the upper arm and the
bone of the forearm lessens

90°

We call this movement **flexion**

180°

Figure 2.6: Flexion of the arm via the contraction of the biceps
muscle (agonist) with the triceps as the potential antagonist.

Flexion and extension are best observed if we view the person performing the movement from the side. *Flexion* is decreasing the angle between two bones connected to the same joint. Let us consider the biceps curl. At rest or at the beginning of the biceps curl, the upper arm and the forearm connected at the elbow joint are at a 180° angle to each other. As we activate the biceps muscles (the muscle performing the desired movement is called the *agonist*), the shortening of their muscle fibers will move the bones of the forearm closer to the bone in the upper arm (in this case, the triceps, for it has the potential of opposing the action of the biceps) the *antagonist* muscle, for it has the potential of opposing the action of the biceps).

Extension is increasing the angle between two bones connected to the same joint. When we perform the chest press, the military press, or do a push-up, we increase the angle between the bones of the upper arm and the forearm by contracting the triceps muscles. During the execution of any of the above exercises resulting in the extension of the arm, the triceps plays the role of the agonist and the biceps the antagonist.

Let us deal briefly with the other movements.

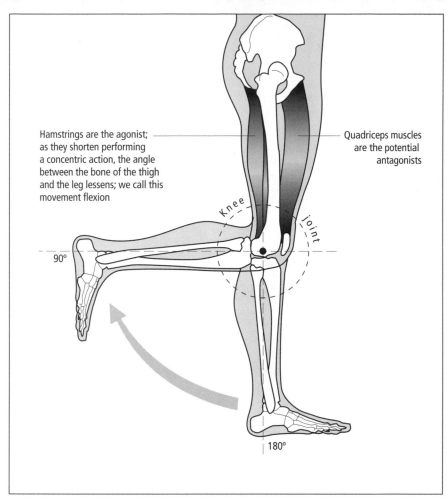

Hamstrings are the agonist; as they shorten performing a concentric action, the angle between the bone of the thigh and the leg lessens; we call this movement flexion

Quadriceps muscles are the potential antagonists

Knee joint

90°

180°

Figure 2.7: Flexion of the leg via the contraction of the hamstrings (agonist) with the quadriceps as the potential antagonist.

Abduction and adduction are best observed by looking at the person performing the movement from the front.

Abduction is a movement away from the midline of the body. When we activate the gluteus medius and gluteus minimus muscles located on the outside region of the hip, they contract as agonists, and the result is the abduction of the thigh. In common language, we lift our leg sidewise, away from the midline of the body, as we view the motion from the front.

Adduction is a movement toward the midline of the body. For example, we sit on a chair with a large exercise ball between our knees. We activate the adductor muscles of the inner thigh and as they contract, we squeeze the exercise ball and both knees move toward the center. When performing this movement, the adductor muscles of the inner thigh play the role of the agonists and the abductor muscles on the lateral region of the hip play the role of the antagonists.

Rotation is the motion of a bone around a central axis. The most frequently rotated bones are the femur at the hip joint and the humerus at the shoulder. Rotating the trunk around the central axis of the spine is also called rotation.

Muscles not only perform movements, they also play an important

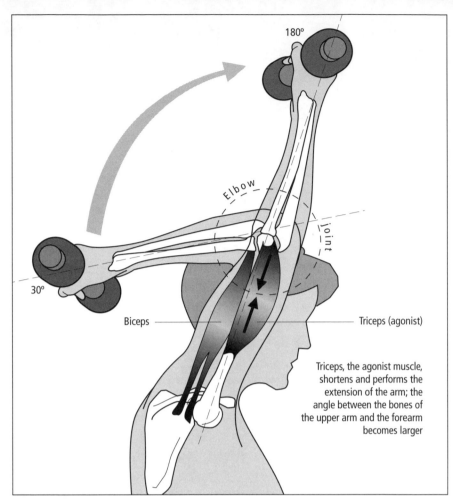

180°

Elbow

joint

30°

Biceps — Triceps (agonist)

Triceps, the agonist muscle, shortens and performs the extension of the arm; the angle between the bones of the upper arm and the forearm becomes larger

Figure 2.8: Extension of the arm via the contraction of the triceps muscle (agonist) with the biceps as the potential antagonist.

part in providing natural and neutral *alignment* of the parts of our body, resulting in healthy *posture*. Some of the most acute and chronic injuries (such as low back pain) are caused by an inability to maintain natural alignment and correct posture due to muscle imbalance.

When exercising, we usually perform one particular exercise several times in order to safely and properly stimulate certain muscle groups.

In exercise terminology, it is called a *repetition* when we perform one prescribed movement. That movement can be flexion, extension, rotation, etc., of a certain body part in relation to another or to the rest of the body. If it is a complicated exercise, it may be a combination of several coordinated movements involving several parts of our bodies.

When we perform more than one repetition of the same movement or a series of movements, it is a *set* of repetitions. If we perform the prescribed movement eight times in a single set, we do a set of eight repetitions. If we perform multiple sets, we might do three sets of eight repetitions.

There are other terms that we will encounter as we read about strength training or have exercise-related conversations in a gym or with our personal trainer.

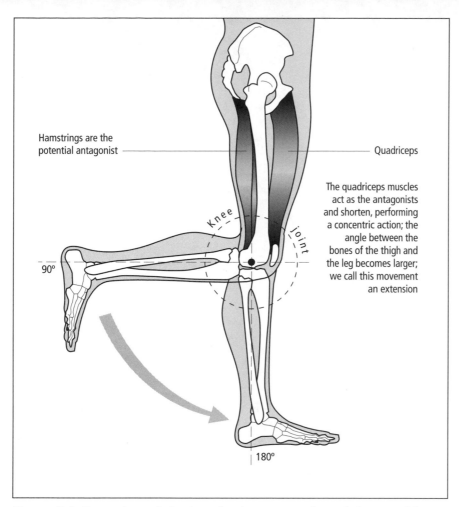

Figure 2.9: Extension of the leg via the contraction of the quadriceps (agonist) with the hamstrings as the potential antagonist.

Muscle fatigue is a temporary phenomenon caused by the depletion of nutrients, lack of sufficient nerve impulse, and an accumulation of lactic acid. Muscle fatigue usually occurs at the end of a set of several repetitions. This temporary muscle fatigue and the accompanying discomfort (burn) usually disappear after a short rest (i.e., about a minute).

Muscle soreness, on the other hand, is a longer-lasting discomfort due to microscopic lesions or tears in the muscle. Depending on the extent of microscopic damage, 48 to 96 hours of rest is needed for the repairs and the rebuilding process, leading to stronger muscles, to be completed.

Muscle strength is the capacity of the muscles to perform a movement against resistance. Maximum strength is the capacity to perform one movement once against maximum resistance. Maximum strength is measured by what is called *one repetition maximum*. I do not recommend that seniors ever test their maximum strength. We are in the business of safely improving, and not dangerously demonstrating our strength.

Muscle endurance is the capacity to perform a certain movement or a series of movements against submaximal resistance several times, usually

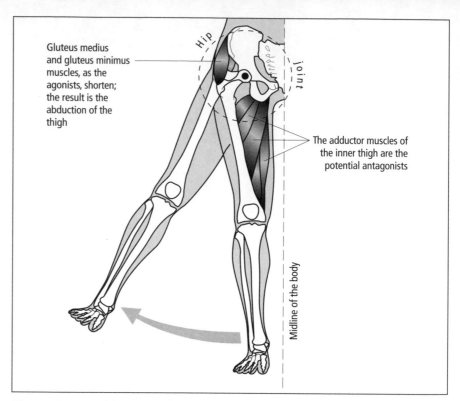

Gluteus medius and gluteus minimus muscles, as the agonists, shorten; the result is the abduction of the thigh

Hip

joint

The adductor muscles of the inner thigh are the potential antagonists

Midline of the body

Figure 2.10: Adduction of the leg via the contraction of the adductor muscles acting as agonists and the gluteus medius and minimus muscles as potential antagonists.

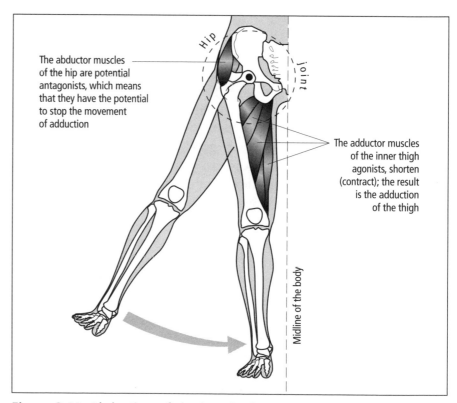

The abductor muscles of the hip are potential antagonists, which means that they have the potential to stop the movement of adduction

Hip

joint

The adductor muscles of the inner thigh agonists, shorten (contract); the result is the adduction of the thigh

Midline of the body

Figure 2.11: Abduction of the leg via the contraction of the gluteus medius and gluteus minimus muscles as agonists with the adductors as potential antagonists.

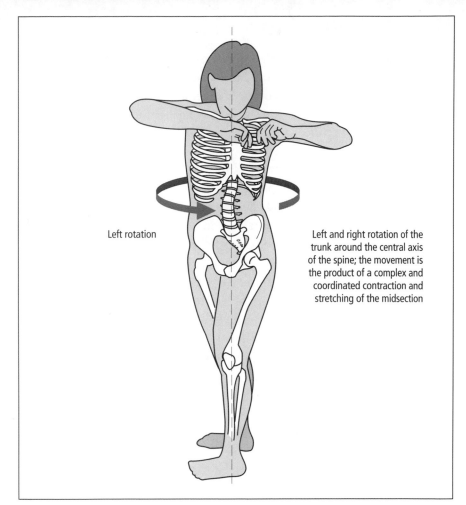

Left rotation

Left and right rotation of the trunk around the central axis of the spine; the movement is the product of a complex and coordinated contraction and stretching of the midsection

Figure 2.12: Rotation of the trunk around the spine

until failure. I also do not recommend that seniors test the limits of their muscle endurance by performing repetitions of an exercise until failure.

Now that we are acquainted with some of the characteristics and function of the human musculature, the biomechanics behind its motions, and have acquired a basic knowledge of the various terms used in the process of strengthening it, we will now proceed to the assessment of our health and fitness level. Without such an assessment, building stronger muscles would be like trying to construct a building without a survey to provide the architect with the initial parameters for drawing a plan.

Health Screening

Most would-be exercisers regard pre-exercise health screening and fitness assessment as unnecessary, tedious, and a waste of time. They cannot be more wrong. The care and attention invested in a thoughtful and sensible gathering of all information relevant to our health and fitness will be rewarded by the benefits of a safe, steady, planned, and successful exercise program.

Health screening and fitness assessment reveals your potential and limitations. This is an integral part of the learning process that allows you to get acquainted with your body. Equipped with the relevant information regarding your health and fitness level, you will be able to avoid injuries, adverse reactions, and serious complications. Without paying due attention to this very important aspect of preparing yourself for a physically active lifestyle, you run the risk of serious injury, may aggravate existing medical conditions, and possibly create unwanted new ones.

It is very important that before you embark on a strength-training program (or any exercise program), you undergo a *health screening* and *fitness assessment* by your family doctor and a qualified fitness professional. The goal of this assessment is to gather and process pertinent information about your medical and fitness status and to identify conditions and medications that may place you at risk when performing certain activities. Without this process of exploration and the resulting conclusions, designing an appropriate strength-training program, setting goals, and planning the pace of progress can be risky and ineffective. Because of age-associated muscle and bone mass reduction, declining flexibility and range of motion, the risk of coronary heart disease, high blood pressure, slow reaction time, loss of balance, and the gradual degradation of many other bodily functions that are greatly aggravated by inactivity, a thorough examination of health and fitness related data is especially important for those who want to begin a strength-training program after a long period of sedentary life.

But regardless of lifestyle habits and chronological age, every senior should get a *medical clearance* and a *fitness assessment* before engaging in strength training or any type of exercise.

Your family doctor, who is familiar with your medical history and the rate of your biological aging, will be able to advise you of the various risks of a strength-training program and provide you with possible contraindications and limitations.

It is also important to check back with your physician after a period of time so that he or she will be able to assess the impact of exercise on your health and suggest modifications in your program, if necessary.

Medications

Several medications may have adverse side effects and older adults are especially vulnerable to not only to adverse side effects, but also to the overall effect of the interaction of drugs, diet, chronic conditions, and exercise.

If you are taking medication, such as anti-hypertensive agents, anti-angina agents, anti-coagulant agents, anti-arrhythmic agents, anti-lipidemic agents, and digitalis glycosides, you should be aware of their side effects in general and specifically as they relate to exercise and how they may influence the body's response to strength training. The side effects may vary from headaches and dizziness to drowsiness and dehydration, and from increased fatigue and bleeding/easy bruising to shortness of breath. They may affect balance, increase or decrease heart rate, or mask fatigue. Your physician will be able to provide you with relevant information regarding this matter and it will influence the nature, amount, and intensity of your strength-training regimen.

What are the most common medical conditions affecting and influencing your exercise program?

- Various forms of cardiovascular diseases—such as coronary artery disease, high blood pressure, heart arrhythmia, or cholesterol levels—that predispose you to cardiovascular diseases
- Various diseases of the kidney, liver, bladder, and digestive tract
- Conditions affecting the nervous system
- Pulmonary and respiratory diseases, such as asthma, bronchitis, and emphysema
- Various forms of degenerative spinal diseases
- Joint diseases, such as arthritis
- Conditions such as sciatica

Each one of the foregoing medical conditions requires special attention and consideration, and each influences the way you or your fitness professional should design and execute your training program.

Fitness Assessment

After obtaining a medical clearance and all the information relevant to your health status, the next step is to have a fitness assessment done by a qualified fitness professional.

There are various ways of obtaining a comprehensive fitness test. Your doctor can arrange for one at a medically approved testing center or clinic. You can also go to a fitness club or to your local for an assessment.

The fitness professional in charge of assessing your fitness status will ask you about your medical history, fitness history, the medications you are presently taking, and various conditions that may affect your ability to exercise. Through practical tests, he or she will check your physical responses to various forms of exercise (aerobic, strength, flexibility tests and gait evaluation). Through various measurements he or she will determine your body composition. *On the basis of a final evaluation of all your medical and fitness data, he or she will be able to recommend an initial exercise program to get you started.*

Once you have acquired a basic knowledge of your musculature and have a pretty good idea of your health and fitness status, the next step is to assess your lifestyle habits and make the necessary adjustments.

When you want to achieve your goal of becoming a stronger and better functioning adult, it is important to assess your lifestyle habits as well as your health and fitness. The positive return for the time and effort invested in improving your strength and fitness will be magnified many times if you adapt lifestyle habits that are conducive to health and fitness. *The two most important healthy lifestyle habits are good nutrition and the ability to cope with stress, including the ability to relax.* Have a critical look at your lifestyle habits, assess them, and, where necessary, make suitable adjustments, otherwise strength training might add another imposition to an already overtaxed system.

There are various methods of achieving positive changes. There are self-declared gurus advocating miraculous methods that they claim will dramatically change everything about you in a few months. That is something that I cannot and will not promise. Rather, I advocate the method that Aristotle recommended when he talked about *arriving at a state of excellence gradually through self-improvement.* He did not look at achieving excellence as one great act, but rather as a series of good, small habits.

In the following pages, we will look at two important components of your general lifestyle. I will explain how they affect your health and fitness. There will be tips on how to make gradual and consistent changes for the better.

Nutrition

If you want to build a strong body, you must give your body quality materials with which to build. Without proper nutrition, you impose an additional demand on your body when you start exercising.

The dominant form of malnutrition in developed societies is *overeating.* Both the volume and the caloric content of the food we eat is more than we need for healthy survival. All-you-can-eat restaurants, colossal servings, and jumbo packaging in supermarkets are the evidence of the popular obsession with quantity, and the excess amount of fat that North Americans carry is the devastating result of this trend. As a result of a combination of overeating, monotonous diet, and lack of activity, by the 1990s, obesity reached endemic proportions among the elderly. The definition of obesity is far from uniform and is measured by various standards. In general, you are considered obese if you are 55–66 lbs (25–30 kg) above the ideal combination of weight and height. Health consequences of obesity range from diabetes to heart disease, from vascular diseases of the brain to flat feet and osteoarthritis of the hips, knees, and lumbar spine. Obesity is associated with high plasma cholesterol, an increased risk of certain cancers, gallbladder disease, and all kinds of psychological problems. For an overweight person, every movement is done at a greater cost and balance is more difficult to maintain. Obese people cannot move quickly, lose coordination, and risk falls and injuries. Accumulation of fat around the abdomen and underneath the diaphragm restricts circulation and breathing. I could go on endlessly about the adverse effects of being obese.[1]

1. Roy J. Shephard, *Aging, Physical Activity and Health* (Champaign, Illinois: Human Kinetics, 1997), p. 274.

Good Nutrition and Stress Management

It is very important that you take a sensible approach to the problem of overeating and a monotonous diet. As I have mentioned earlier, *setting realistic goals, achieving gradual improvements, and enjoying the process of achieving them is more conducive to lasting results than dramatic and desperate actions* that usually lead to frustration, disappointment, and, finally, to defeat.

Look at what you eat and decide which foods should be eliminated from your diet and which should be introduced into it. Be persistent. Make a list and work on that list patiently and gradually. Keep a record of what you eat. Make reasonable decisions based on readily available and proven facts and current nutrition science. *Enjoy the process of becoming a healthy eater instead of suddenly embracing one fad or the other.* If in doubt, hire a reputable, certified nutritionist.

In the following pages, I will give a few examples of what and how I eat. Use it as a guide to a healthy diet.

I usually eat some fiber-rich, wholesome cereal in the morning. There are hundreds of cereals packaged in attractive boxes and some of them have no more value than the box they are sold in. They usually contain some form of processed and denaturalized grain, sugar, artificial flavor and color, and other additives. However, there are a number of healthy and nutritious cereals, rich in fibers and low in sugar and other additives, now available. Without advocating any brand, my favorites are the Ancient Grains™, Seven Grains™, and Multigrain™ and Fibre First Multi-Bran™ from President's Choice and All-Bran Buds™ from Kellogg's. There are also other wholesome cereals from other manufacturers. I like to add blueberries, papaya, strawberries, or raspberries and either skim milk or soy milk to my cereal.

Another breakfast I like is no-fat, plain yogurt with papaya, strawberries, blueberries, and/or raspberries. Sometimes I eat scrambled eggs with lots of green pepper, tomato, and onion and whole-wheat bread. If I use three eggs, I take the yolk out of two. I always drink some green tea in the morning. After breakfast, I prepare my snacks for the day. I put celery stalks, carrots, diced turnips, and sprouts into a sealable bag, and almonds, walnuts, sunflower seeds, and pumpkin seeds in another.

I also juice celery, turnips, cucumbers, and beets and put the vegetable juice in a bottle and add some ground flaxseed. I call this "Metabolic Dominance" for I am confident that this strange brew helped me win nine world titles in various master events from kayaking to a quadrathlon. In 1999 I won the master category in the Diamond Man Long-Distance Quadrathlon Worlds (5k swim, 20k kayak, 100k bike, and 21k run) in Ibiza, Spain. After I finished, I was celebrating with my friends when the relay team of the British Royal Marines came in to finish their race. They were all in their twenties, and as it was a relay, they had a swimmer, a kayaker, a biker, and a runner. I finished the race solo about two minutes ahead of them. I was drinking my "Metabolic Dominance" when one of them came up to me and asked me how it was possible that I could beat them. "I drink swamp juice," I said and offered my bottle of juiced celery, beets, carrots, and turnips with ground flaxseed. They tasted it and decided they liked Coke™ better. Next year I beat them by four minutes and that converted two of them to my "Metabolic Dominance."

Throughout the morning I snack on my seeds and greens and drink my swamp juice until lunchtime. For lunch I eat grilled chicken, fish, or turkey with steamed broccoli, green peas, green beans, and yams, after which I snack until dinner. I have my dinner early and eat lightly. It is usually some green salad with tofu, olive oil, and lemon juice.

Besides looking at *what* you eat, you might also want to look at *how* you eat. I always eat relatively little at any one time. I also try to eat slowly. I chew my food well—digestion starts in the mouth. If I eat quickly, the message to the brain indicating that I have eaten enough is usually late and, before it registers, I have already overeaten. I also try to reduce the amount of what I eat before going to bed.

There is nothing magical about my diet. My philosophy is quite simple. I like eating good, wholesome foods because I know that they are an important factor in my health and fitness, and I prefer health and fitness to illness. I do not overeat because I like to be lean and slim a lot more than being obese and fat. I stay away from the attraction of easily available bad food because I know that the price I pay for giving in to the temptation of taste and convenience will be high. I do not fall for fads because the bogus science they are based on does not make any sense to me.

Of course, there are people who, for one reason or another, need a more regulated and stricter regimen in the form of a reasonable diet prescribed by a qualified nutritionist. If you choose this venue, you will be required to follow that regimen and keep a record of what and how much you eat, which is a good idea.

If you cannot afford the services of a registered nutritionist, you may want to go for such diets as the one advocated by Dr. Dean Ornish, or choose a reasonable popular diet such as the South Beach Diet (books on both are available in your local bookstore). *Stay away from fads and charlatans who promise spectacular and dramatic changes, but fail to inform you about the health costs and the impossibility of maintaining the changes in the long term.* Do not listen to pseudoscientific humbug recommending the elimination of carbohydrates from your diet. There are good complex carbohydrates low on the glycemic index—such as beans, lentils, chickpeas, barley, legumes, nuts, seeds, and whole-wheat multigrain bakery products—that slowly and gradually diffuse energy throughout the body.

The glycemic index is a ranking of carbohydrates according to their immediate effect on blood glucose (blood sugar) levels. Carbohydrates that break down quickly during digestion have the highest glycemic ratings. The blood glucose response to these carbs is fast and high. Carbohydrates that break down slowly, releasing glucose gradually into the bloodstream, have low glycemic ratings.

- Low GI means a less significant rise in blood glucose levels after meals
- Low GI diets help lose weight

- Low GI foods can improve the body's sensitivity to insulin
- Low GI diet can improve diabetes control
- Low GI foods keep you feeling full longer
- Low GI foods can prolong physical endurance
- Glycemic index range:
  - Low GI = 55 or less
  - Medium GI = 55–69
  - High GI = 70 or more

The same goes for no-fat diets. There are essential fatty acids in deep-sea fish oil, flaxseed oil, etc., that are absolutely necessary for maintaining a healthy body.

The most effective way to improve your eating habits is to gradually eliminate bad food and gradually introduce more wholesome foods into your diet.

Eliminate:

- saturated fats and trans-fats
- hydrogenated oils
- soft drinks/sodas
- sweets and candies

Drastically reduce:

- processed foods
- red meat
- salt
- simple carbohydrates that are high on the glycemic index, such as dates, fruit rolls, waffles, white bagels, doughnuts, french fries, cornflakes, corn syrup, honey, and potatoes
- alcohol

Introduce:

- dark green leafy vegetables, such as spinach, chard, etc.
- cruciferous vegetables, such as bok choy, broccoli, Brussel sprouts, cabbage, cauliflower, collards, kale, kohlrabi, rutabaga, turnip greens, and turnip, etc.
- sprouts
- hummus
- fresh vegetable juices
- seeds and nuts
- legumes such as lentils, peas, beans, etc.
- fruit such as berries, papaya, apple, apricot, watermelon, citrus
- healthy oils such as omega-3 oils found in fish oils and flaxseed oil
- protein-rich, healthy foods such as tofu, fish, turkey, soy products, and egg whites
- skimmed milk products such as no-fat plain yogurt

Bad habits such as smoking, drinking, and consuming products that contain caffeine also interfere with your goal of getting fitter.

In addition to overeating, another common form of malnutrition is a monotonous diet. This means that the food we eat is not only too much in quantity and too rich in empty calories, but at the same time lacks quality, variety, and balance and is deficient in vitamins, minerals, fibers, and essential fatty acids.

It is common knowledge that processed foods are devoid of healthy nutrients and loaded with preservatives, coloring, and taste-enhancing agents that are not just a source of empty calories but may be harmful to your health. Processed foods are not only dead—that is, lacking in natural vitamins, minerals, and essential fatty acids—but may be toxic as well. By toxic, I do not mean that they contain poisons that kill you in days, but if they are habitually eaten over a long period, they may lead to chronic bad health. It is a fact that excess consumption of processed sugar (the most commonly used additive and preservative) causes, among other illnesses, diabetes. Another common additive, salt, causes high blood pressure by stiffening the walls of blood vessels. What makes excess sugar and salt very dangerous to your health is that they are present in all processed and canned food. Most of us do not know that just one can of chicken noodle soup (or two pickled cucumbers) contains the total daily recommended intake of salt. Then there are the myriad chemicals added to processed foods to prevent them from drying, aging, turning hard, changing color, etc.

Another problem with processed foods is that they provide a dreary, uniform diet. Processed foods are degermed and heat-treated, stabilized and converted. Natural fibers, enzymes, and important phytochemicals are removed. In short, most processed foods are denaturalized. They provide easily available empty calories that play havoc with your blood sugar, make you bloated, overweight, clog up your system, and fail to give you the vigor and vitality needed to resist diseases. The number one step you should take on your way to a healthier life is to slowly but consistently reduce the amount of processed foods you eat. You cannot exclude everything, but you can do a pretty good job in eliminating the worst.

The best way to reduce obesity and improve body composition is to combine exercise and good eating habits. A well-designed physical activity program accompanied by improvements in your eating habits will work better than either exercise or diet alone. Attention to good eating habits will provide all the quality building materials for the exerciser to build a fit and healthy body, and exercise will ensure that the food is used for better and more effective functions and not deposited as fat, plaque, and undesirable accumulation of waste products and bodily fluids. It has been proven that among the many metabolic effects of exercise, regular physical activity can enhance protein synthesis, speed up gastrointestinal transit time, elevate basal metabolic rate, and promote the absorption of vitamins and minerals. The overall effect is a loss of fat and a gain in lean, functional muscle mass.

Besides gradually improving my eating habits over several years, I also acquired good habits and skills that help me achieve and maintain a healthy mind and a healthy body. I find that my ability to cope with stress and my capacity to relax are a very important part of my overall strategy for health and fitness.

Stress Management

You might have been able to ignore the signals and suppress some of the manifestations of stress and function normally to a certain degree in your life, but generally at around age 50, you begin to pay the price of the cumulative effects of stress.

In his famous book, *The Stress of Life*, Hans Selye, who coined the word "stress" and founded the Canadian Institute of Stress, describes stress as a complex chain of internal reactions that occur when we perceive a threat to our existence or well-being. *Excessive stress occurs when the level of aggravation exceeds our capacity to absorb and to deal with the demands imposed upon us.*

Stress had its role in evolution when early human beings had to confront all kinds of physical danger. It was part of the fight-or-flight response: the brain suddenly focused on the threat. Forgetting everything else, the heart began to beat faster, adrenalin was pumped into the blood, arteries suddenly dilated, and stored energy supplies were rapidly mobilized as the body went on high alert. Fear for our physical survival has long since been replaced by fear of losing control.

The salient stressors in our lives today, generally in developed societies, are mental/emotional. They come mostly from our interactions with people or in dealing with situations in which we perceive that we have little or no control. They can be mentally challenging if we can respond to them healthily and effectively, but they can also be threatening and overwhelming if we perceive them as such. These stressors and the psychological stress they create affect our health and well-being in many ways. *The impact of psychological stress and the resulting negative emotions affect not only our nervous system in the form of nervous agitation/irritation, depression, and anxiety but also the behavior of almost every cell in our bodies.* It destabilizes the body's homeostasis, upsets biological chemical balances, and disrupts our entire system. As a result, the healthy functioning of the whole body degrades. If the amount, duration, and intensity of stress are more than we can absorb and react to in a healthy manner, the consequences may range from headaches to ulcers, from depression to alcohol and drug abuse, from the repression of our immune system to high blood pressure and heart disease. The negative reactions to cumulative stress may manifest themselves in flare-ups of rheumatoid arthritis, fat deposits around the abdomen, a disruption of the delicate balance between the brain and the endocrine system that makes and releases hormones, and in the release of harmful compounds that cause inflammation. In short, *stress reduces our strength and ability to maintain a healthy physique.*

The problem is that we can have anxiety, depression, and physical symptoms as a result of prolonged and unabated stress without any obvious sense of discomfort. For some of us, stress has been such a constant, unremitting fact of daily life that we do not even recognize it as one of the most dangerous and harmful attacks on our well-being. This inability to recognize and to be aware of what is happening to us may lead us to take on extra stress instead of trying to find a way to cope with it in a healthy and effective manner. At a certain point in our lives, *the cumulative effect of stress on body and mind will become so overwhelming that almost any negative experience can start a full avalanche of adverse reactions* and we may find ourselves vulnerable to a variety of mental and physical ailments.

We cannot avoid all the stressors in our daily lives. However, we can develop skills to cope with them so that they will not play havoc with our mental/emotional and physical well-being by creating a bizarre civil war between an unbalanced mind and a weak body.

The timely recognition of stress signals and destructive patterns is the most important first step in dealing with stress. Without this recognition and the resulting awareness, there is no action we can take and we remain vulnerable to life's stresses.

These are the emotional signs we may experience when stress overwhelms us:

- irrational fear
- irritation
- anger
- worrying
- nervousness
- loss of sense of humor
- general negativity
- emotional exhaustion
- instability
- lethargy
- depression

These are the changes we may observe in our overt behavior under excess stress:

- pacing and talking to ourselves or arguing
- overeating and rushed eating or loss of appetite
- shaky hands
- missed appointments
- swearing
- negative self-talk
- outbursts of anger
- nagging others
- sudden increase in bad habits such as smoking, or drinking alcohol and caffeine
- a desire to work more and an increase in the number of mistakes while working
- withdrawing, avoiding others, and wanting to be alone

Physical signs:

- tightness in the neck and shoulders, throat, and chest
- slumped posture
- headaches
- strained face
- shaky hands
- sweating
- rapid and shallow breathing
- dry mouth
- physical weakness
- skin rashes

The second step is to identify the causes of stress or stressors that elicit adverse reactions and deal with them appropriately. Among the most common sources of stress are personal ambitions, perceptions, unreasonable expectations, preoccupations, and overreaching and resulting loss of control.

It is not easy to identify these sources because it takes self-knowledge, the ability to admit that *most of the time I am not a passive sufferer, but an active promoter of stress.* This admission logically requires that I take action and modify or eliminate certain behavioral patterns that work against my own well-being. I might have little faith in my ability to do that. I might also have to seek advice and I would regard it as an admission of weakness. What I would most likely do is ignore and try to further repress my symptoms, much as the character in a Woody Allen movie who proudly proclaims that he never shows anger. He grows ulcers instead.

I learned that instead of ignoring and repressing the symptoms, I should listen carefully to my body and improve my personal skills to deal with stress. Stressors do not go away, and symptoms cannot be endlessly repressed. I must find ways of coping with them. I was past 55 when I acquired the proper mindset and tools to cope with life's stresses. Let us talk about the mindset first.

Positive mindset is an effective and established system of conscious control of my mental/emotional processes to the advantage of my well-being.

Negative mindset is the lack of such an established system or the presence or existence of a system that works against my own well-being.

I recognized that without conscious control, I am a wavering creature of moods, easily thrown off judgment and purpose, a specialist in misunderstanding. Without conscious control, my reactions are reflex-like, impulsive, and counterproductive. I get easily preoccupied with useless thoughts and emotions, and am resigned to irrational, undesirable, and counterproductive behavioral patterns. Without conscious control, I enhance my weaknesses instead of reducing them. The end result is defeat and capitulation to life's stresses.

Fortunately, I also recognized that if I persist in patiently adjusting my mindset in the direction of the positive and keep strengthening, conditioning, and honing it, I have a pretty good chance at meeting the challenges of life's stresses. From experience, I learned that a *positive mindset is the most powerful conscious force I can have in regulating the way I use my energy so that it benefits myself and others.* What are the qualities that make one's mindset positive?

The ability to:

- think in a calm, pacified, and reflective manner instead of being disturbed, agitated, and impulsive in reactions
- put ideas together rationally and arrive at the right judgment even in the absence of obvious evidence or proof
- decide, plan, and execute a course of action in a patient, persistent, and disciplined manner
- recognize changes and be flexible in adapting to them
- observe and perceive things with a sense of humor instead of outrage, indignation, and anger
- let go instead of being preoccupied with useless and counterproductive thoughts, desires, and ambitions
- relax and meditate or rest
- resist temptation and coercion

Do I have a mindset that is characterized by all these qualities? Certainly not, but by trial and error, by falling on my face and getting up again, I constantly improve my mindset.

What are the practical skills and tools and the mental processes that I use in coping with stress in a positive way? With practice and patience, everyone can develop and then enjoy the command of his or her own technique for dealing with stress.

The most readily available and easiest to use tool in my toolbox is breathing. As soon as I feel worry, tension, anxiety, anger, or any other negative feeling, I start deep, abdominal breathing—I inhale deeply and hold my breath for a few moments. Then I exhale fully and stretch my diaphragm by expanding the chest without inhaling for another few moments. Then I do another deep, abdominal inhale. I completely focus on this breathing exercise, trying to increase the volume of air I inhale to the maximum and trying to exhale fully.

I use breathing regularly to calm my mind and my senses. I do breathing exercises at least six or seven times daily. I find it calming, relaxing, and energizing. I do this exercise before my races. I always deep-breathe when I walk. It is the perfect combination of aerobic exercise and relaxation.

Breathing exercises not only calm my mind, but make it almost impossible to be anxious while breathing deeply and holding both the inhale and the exhale for a few moments. Besides mental relaxation, deep breathing also helps lower blood pressure, and improves circulation and digestion.

I have a particular breathing exercise for each stressor. Someone recently asked me how I handle stress, and I answered that I have special breathing exercises for it. When he looked at me incredulously, I jokingly added that I have about 20 different breathing exercises to cope with my

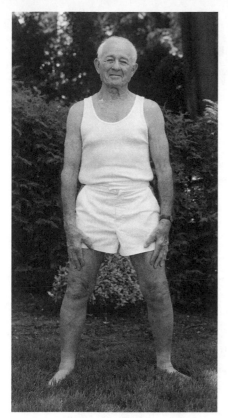 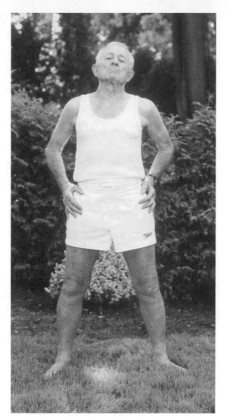 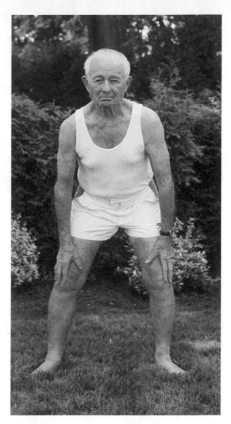

Starting Position: Stand with your feet shoulder width apart and with your arms in a relaxed, extended position. the palms of your hands should gently touch the sides of your thighs.

Inhale: Begin inhaling slowly. First into the abdomen than into the chest. At the final stage of the inhale, expand and lift the chest as much as you can. You can assist the expansion of the ribcage by pressing your hands against your thighs. Hold breath for a few moments.

Exhale: Begin exhaling by slowly contracting the abdominal muscles and compressing the chest. At the final phase of the exhale lean forward and rest your hand above your knees.

family, including myself. In fact, out of that 20, at least 10 help me tolerate myself.

My second way of dealing with stress is rest. I have the tendency to run all day and work on various projects until I drop, so I accumulate such a deficit of sleep and rest that it seriously affects my well-being. I have to focus on slowing myself down, and the best way to do it is to have one siesta during my working day. I do some breathing exercises, then lie on the floor with my feet on an exercise ball and slowly park my thoughts until I can relax and rest for about half an hour.

My third tool is using small, sensible solutions to problems and situations that I cannot avoid or tolerate. Here are a few examples:

- I do not like to wait, so I always carry a book with me to read.
- I do not like to be stuck in traffic, so I have a collection of classical music to play in the car when it happens.
- I always carry a notebook because I tend to forget things and then get upset about it.

We all grow older, but it is by no means certain that we will all grow up. Some of us cannot get rid of the childish tendency to believe that life conspires to make us happy or miserable. This immature pattern of thinking can follow us well into old age and leads to unnecessary aggravation. It took me some time to grow up and admit and accept that some things just happen.

Among the mental processes I use to cope with stress is to adjust my perception so that things that appear threatening, insulting, unreasonable, and in some way or another directed at me are consciously interpreted as funny, silly, incidental, and something to laugh at. I look them with a sense of humor. I look for a reason to smile, laugh, or just quietly amuse myself instead of being outraged, indignant, insulted, and threatened.

With conscious control, I am able to adjust my perception and can overcome the compulsion to react at all. I reflect instead. I used to respond immediately to every proposal, question, or provocation with agreement or disagreement. Now I feel free to say that I do not know and I will have to think about it. I also feel free to ignore whatever I find unreasonable or inappropriate or both.

I never try to be perfect. I always try to do the best I can under the circumstances, but I am not obsessed by the desire to be perfect. I do not expect others and the world to be perfect either. I look at greater perfection as something I work toward and I enjoy the process of improving myself, but never entertain the illusion that I will ever achieve perfection.

Because this book is about strength training, I do not want to deal more than necessary with the importance of stress management. At the same time, I cannot emphasize enough that *without exercising the mind and training it to cope with stress, one cannot realize half of one's potential to become physically stronger.*

At this point, you have acquired a basic knowledge of the human musculature. You are cleared by your doctor and assessed by a fitness professional. You also know that good nutrition and healthy lifestyle habits are just as important as physical training for your well-being.

The next step is to set realistic and achievable goals that are also challenging and motivating. In the next chapter, we will deal with the importance of goal setting.

BEHAVIOR-Change Commitment Contract

1. I, Mighty Senior, will begin my behavior-change program immediately and will incorporate the following into my daily routine.

2. I will pay attention to and try to recognize physical, behavioral, and mental/emotional signs of stress and be aware of these signs. I will record common adverse reactions to stress, which may include everything from overeating to negative feelings.

3. I will try to identify the sources of stress and be aware of them.

4. I will steadily work on improving my personal skills to cope with stress that results in fear, impulsiveness, anxiety, anger, preoccupation, and other negative feelings by:
   (a) working on building a positive mindset that includes changing perceptions, reactions, and being more reflective rather than reactive
   (b) using breathing, relaxing, meditating, reading, listening to music, etc., to prevent and cope with stress
   (c) constantly reviewing and appreciating the progress I am making and rewarding myself
   (d) enlisting the services of a professional counselor if I need outside support to do all the above

April 12, 2005   Mighty Senior

_____   _____
DATE   SIGNATURE

Note: You will find a blank copy of this form at the end of this book.

Stress Management Strategies

1. I listen to what my body is telling me:
   a. tightness
   b. slumped posture
   c. shaky hands
   d. sweating and night sweating
   e. headaches
   f. dry mouth
   g. rapid and shallow breathing
   h. lack of energy
   i. strained face

2. I am aware of the following behavioral signals and their sources:

Signal	Identify Source
Talking to myself/arguing	_____
Overeating/rushed eating	_____
Swearing	_____
Outbursts of anger	_____
Nagging others	_____
Increase in bad habits	_____
Withdrawing	_____
Working more and making mistakes	_____

3. Emotional signs:

Signal	Identify Source
a. fear	_____
b. anger	_____
c. worrying	_____
d. loss of sense of humor	_____
e. irritation	_____

4. I employ the following strategies to manage my stress:
   a. Change my perception of things; acquire a sense of humor
   b. Reduce ambitions/lower expectations/become more realistic and accepting
   c. Learn to say no
   d. Get adequate sleep and rest
   e. Do breathing and various relaxation techniques
   f. Seek counsel

Note: You will find a blank copy of this form at the end of this book.

Behavioral Balance Sheet

Under the "Comments" columns, note when you feel each emotion.

Positive	Comments	Negative	Comments
1. Sense of humor	e.g., I laugh at myself when I make a mistake.	1. Fear	e.g., I feel fear when I have to go for checkup.
2. Calmness		2. Anxiety	
3. Ability to reflect		3. Nervousness	
4. Ability to say no		4. Outrage	
5. Assertiveness		5. Indignation	
6. Optimism		6. Preoccupation	
7. Patience		7. Impatience	
8. Discipline		8. Pessimism	
9. Awareness		9. Annoyance	
10. Ability to let go		10. Worrying	

Note: You will find a blank copy of this form at the end of this book.

We seem to set mental limits on the possible boundaries of our world and work within these limits.[1] We tend to be resigned to what we are and what we can do. At the same time, we are also able to imagine ourselves in the pursuit of a goal, and have the capacity to plan how to attain it.

We have a choice. We can either behave passively *or* we can be proactive in making ourselves what we want to be.

When you decide to embark on a healthy and physically active life, you must set realistic and reasonable goals. To achieve these goals, you devise a game plan, a process based on a method.

By nature, we humans are motivated by goals. Mentally and emotionally we want an improved existence, a greater perfection that we have visualized and imagined. Our whole conscious life is based on setting our sights on a goal or a set of goals and organizing our activities toward achieving them.

Without goals, our actions lack concreteness, direction, and focus. Positive attitudes will fade away, discipline will slowly erode, commitment becomes less firm, the temptation to give up will prevail over the motivation to continue, and a fear of failure will win over our determination to succeed.

A sensible goal is a realistic target that we consciously aim to reach and accomplish. Once it has been set, we must remain committed to it. It will be the purpose of our actions, of what we do in a disciplined, intelligent, and consistent manner. We cannot overestimate the psychological/inspirational value of realistic short- and long-term goals in providing the training process with direction, focus, consistency, and stability.

It is very important that on the basis of our health and fitness status, we set realistic short- and long-term goals for ourselves. *These goals must be difficult enough to challenge us, but must be realistic to be achievable.* We must be convinced that the price of goals—that is, the time, effort, and care we invest in achieving them—is worthwhile and that the goals will eventually lead us to a better quality of life, more fun, enjoyment, and independence.

When it comes to strength fitness, short- and long-term goals are different for each person. Whatever the goals are, we need motivating, concrete, and precise goals that can be as simple as getting up from a chair without assistance or as challenging as being a champion master athlete. In some cases, at the beginning, the goal is to perform some basic functions better and may progress into truly exceptional performances. I have had several elderly clients (who now would vehemently resent the description "elderly") whose initial goals were to perform basic functions. Before they knew it, they went from being sedentary to gradually accomplishing quite spectacular performances and became master swimmers, kayakers, canoeists, and triathletes. It is impossible to give a complete list of personalized goals in a book. The idea is to start with simple, realistic, and achievable goals and raise the standard gradually and sensibly. What is most important is enjoying the step-by-step process of achieving our goals.

1. R.E. Orstein, *The Psychology of Consciousness* (New York: Penguin Books, 1986), p. 1.

As I mentioned before, goals will encourage a positive attitude in us, and will provide stronger motivation, firmer commitment, better discipline, sharper focus, patience and perseverance. Let us deal separately with each of these.

The ability to make an intelligent and consistent effort and the ability to resist temptation to give up is a positive attitude. Goals inspire a positive attitude in us. They draw us and move us toward where we want to be and inspire us to go on. Goals help us overcome inertia, fear, and the inability to act.

Motivation

Motivation is the inner drive, the impulse that makes us act. Motivation is the power that produces action and motion. It is the inner force that provides the mental/emotional energy, the impetus to act. Some people lack motivation—no energy, momentum, inclination, or incentive to get going—and are inactive or passive. *Setting goals and visualizing yourself achieving your goals will help you get moving and will give you the mental impetus and energy to act.*

Some may have a certain amount of drive, but that drive may lack commitment, discipline, focus, and direction. It might be vague, dispersed, and misdirected. Blind drive is not conducive to success. Rather, it leads to frustration, failure, and defeat. *In order to be successful in our endeavors, our drive and motivation need a strong commitment, focus, discipline, and direction.* It is not enough to get excited and enthusiastic about something. It is true that without motivation we would not be attracted to the idea of fitness, but without serious commitment, discipline, and focus, motivation will not last long. Goals help to maintain the level of motivation, commitment, discipline, focus, patience, and persistence needed to stay on track.

Commitment

Commitment is the act of making up your mind, pledging yourself to a cause, embracing a course, and engaging yourself in something.

Once we set our sight on a goal, we must make a commitment to take a measured, decisive, and immediate action to achieve it. The longer you postpone committing yourself, the more you behave like the legendary fisherman who decided to wait for the ocean to drain away so that he can collect his fish. But the ocean (in this case, excuses) will be there forever.

When it comes to training, commitment is the amount of time, effort, patience, persistence, discipline, and hard work that you are prepared to dedicate toward achieving your goal. Among the most important strategies that increase your likelihood of success is commitment. It is the starting point for the realization of goals.

During the process of achieving your goals, you must constantly foster, maintain, and increase your level of commitment, for it is the psychological foundation on which training, achievement, and success is built.

Discipline

Discipline is the glue that holds our thinking and actions together. Without discipline, neither our thinking nor actions have organization, cohesion, direction, or focus. The term "discipline" comes from the Latin word *disciplina* and means training for order, self-control, and efficiency of action according to a system of proven methods. *You will achieve your goals only if you follow the rules of training without compromise.* Any laxity or lack of care and concern will make you a plaything of your mood and inclination. Your workouts will be irregular, your progression erratic, and the result will be failure and defeat.

Focus

Focus is the uninterrupted connection between you and something that you do. It can make the difference in performing the exercises correctly with good form, good posture, and good breathing. The ability to focus makes it possible to be absorbed in the movement, blocking out any distracting thoughts and emotions. The ability to seek, find, hold onto, and be absorbed in the feel of the movement adds quality to your exercises. Without focus, you just go through the motions without proper attention to coordination, range of motion, or fluidity of movements. The exercise you perform may make your muscles stronger, but because there will be no quality to the exercise, it will have little functional value.

Patience and Persistence

The ability to be patient and persevere without losing interest or heart before things work out in your favor is absolutely necessary to achieve your goals. If you are impatient and want immediate results, you will rush and fail to pay due attention to correct form, correct posture, correct breathing, and gradual progression. You will risk injuries and burnouts. Alternatively, you may observe the rules of training, but in your impatience to reach your goals, you exercise a lot more and more frequently than your body is able to absorb and adapt to. Although you might achieve your first goal sooner, your body will be unable to keep up with the demands imposed on it and you will fail to achieve your long-term goals. Frustrated and defeated, you will lose heart before you can enjoy the benefits of your efforts. Setting realistic short-term and long-term goals and enjoying the process of achieving them will teach you how to be patient and persistent.

Goals can range from wanting to be able to climb stairs to being able to canoe down the Hood River in Canada's arctic. Some may want to get into a dress of a certain size or look good in a swimsuit. *Whatever your goal, it will enhance motivation, commitment, discipline, focus, patience, and persistence.* A lack of realistic short- and long-term goals will slowly erode motivation, commitment, and discipline. Setting and pursuing unrealistic goals will lead to disappointment, failure, and defeat. The trick is to have a pretty good idea of your present health and fitness status, your abilities and potentials, and establish your goals so that they will be a challenge and a roadmap.

The general, long-term goal of strength training is to become stronger. In order to progress consistently, we need to commit ourselves to a few initial short-term goals that are achievable within two or three months. *These short-term goals must be specific, measurable, attainable, relevant, and time-bound.*

A commitment contract, in which we briefly outline the initial goals of the next two or three months and our ways of achieving them, is a very important part of our success strategy. It is also important to daily reaffirm our belief in our ability to reach these initial goals.

Let us say, for example, that you are about 25 lbs (11 kg) overweight. You eat too much red meat, too much processed foods, and sugars in the form of sweets. You can perform five parallel squats with your body weight and five biceps curls with a 10 lb (4.5 kg) dumbbell. You have a problem coping with stress and are easily angered.

In your commitment contract (see the contract at the end of the chapter), after assessing your eating habits, you pledge to lose 10 lbs (4.5 kg) in three months by reducing your consumption of red meat, processed foods, and sweets and by increasing the amount of fresh green vegetables, fiber-rich foods, and skimmed milk products.

You pledge to strength train three times a week, for forty-five minutes each time, according to a comprehensive program of lower-body, trunk, and upper-body exercises. Your goal is to perform ten parallel squats with your body weight and twelve biceps curls with a 10 lb (4.5 kg) dumbbell.

Through breathing exercises and other suitable coping and relaxing strategies such as walking, meditating, and resting, instead of suppressing, you learn to diffuse and prevent potential angry reactions.

These realistic short-term goals will complement each other. Eating wholesome foods that are less in calories but higher in nutritional value will help you lose weight and provide better quality material for building lean muscles. More lean muscles will increase your basal metabolic rate and you will burn more calories even at rest. Losing weight will make it easier for you to do squats with your own body weight, making exercising more pleasurable. Breathing exercises, relaxation, and the resulting ability to cope with stress will free up energies that would be otherwise wasted and dispersed by negative emotions such as anger, and redirect those energies toward achieving your goals.

The achievement of these short-term goals will also inspire you to visualize your long-term goals. The self-knowledge you gain during the process will enable you to be more precise in detailing your long-term goals.

If you could lose 10 lbs (4.5 kg) in three months, it is reasonable to plan to lose 25 lbs (11 kg) in a year. (Try not to assume that the initial pace of progress can be or should be maintained forever.) With a stronger and lighter body fuelled by wholesome food of better quality, you can set your sights more precisely at various improvements in lower-, torso, and upper-body strength. With improved skills in coping with stress, you may also want to widen the scope of your training by participating in various recreational or competitive activities. These long-term goals can be revised and adjusted according to your rate of progress and health status.

An Exercise/Lifestyle Commitment Contract

I, Mighty Senior, pledge that I shall commit to the following:

- I shall do strength training three times a week on the following non-consecutive days: Monday, Wednesday, and Friday.

- I shall adhere to the proper procedures of strength training, including proper warm-up, correct execution of exercises, stretching, and cool-down.

- I shall walk at least 30 minutes daily at a brisk pace to improve and maintain my cardiovascular fitness.

- In order to maximize my improvements and to fully realize my potential, I shall systematically improve my lifestyle habits, such as nutrition and stress management, practise breathing exercises twice a day, and give myself opportunities to relax.

- My short-term goals for the next three months are the following:

  a. Lose *15 lbs (7 kg)*.

  b. Be able to *complete a set of 12 half squats*.

  c. Be able to *complete a set of 12 wall push-ups*.

- My long-term goals for the year are the following:

  a. Lose *30 lbs (14 kg)*.

  b. Lower my blood pressure to *normal*.

  c. Be able to *complete a set of 12 half squats with ten 10 lb (4.5 kg) dumbbells*.

  d. Be able to *complete a set of 12 dumbbell bench presses with 15 lbs (7 kg)*.

  e. Be able to *hike for two hours on a trail*.

- I shall keep a daily journal of my activities.

- I shall daily affirm my commitment to do all the above.

- I shall find ways of rewarding myself for every improvement.

April 12, 2005   Mighty Senior

_____   _____
DATE   SIGNATURE

Note: You will find a blank copy of this form at the end of this book.

You will experience irregular, short-lived improvements in your strength by following almost any strength-training program. Some popular programs may result in spectacular, short-term gains, but usually carry a high risk of injuries and burnouts. Gains in muscle strength are rarely balanced and almost never translated into functional skills. Some other popular programs are too general in order to be effective and fail to provide a reasonable rate of improvement.

In order to meet our requirements, a well-designed training program for seniors must be:

1. *Safe:* The program must be designed and executed so that the potential for injuries and the likelihood of aggravating existing medical conditions or creating new ones are minimal.

2. *Effective:* The training program has to be designed, executed, and constantly adjusted so that *it produces the best possible results.* It must remain challenging and stimulating without straining the body. The amount, intensity, and complexity of the workouts, interspersed with the proper amount of rest (recovery) and with periods of consolidation—that is, when we slow down or cease progression and firmly establish the results achieved—must be manipulated so that the result will be a steady and optimal gain in muscle strength.

3. *Personalized: It must take into account the specific needs of the individual,* such as health and fitness status, biological age, potential, and short- and long-term goals and aspirations.

4. *Functional: It must translate the improvements in muscle strength into real-life functional capabilities.*

5. *Progressive: It must ensure that there is progress toward your goals.* Once certain gains are achieved and firmly established, further improvements are targeted. There is always something to be improved—from coordination to posture, from flexibility to muscle endurance.

6. *Balanced: It must develop the musculature in a balanced and proportionate manner.* It must also balance several other aspects of fitness, such as posture, flexibility, and gait.

Safe

You have acquainted yourself with the basics of human anatomy, and the location and workings of your musculature. After careful consideration, you design your initial training program based on your medical history, fitness assessment, biological age, and activity level. You take into account the level of your physical skills, including coordination, reaction time, sense of balance, and speed of movement. *Finding the optimal exercises, the optimal workload, and the optimal rate of progression will still be by trial and error.*

Injuries and the possibility of aggravating existing medical conditions or creating new ones may not only stop you from continuing training, but may also seriously affect your health, so *it is wise to be cautious* when you embark on your strength-training program.

Select the exercises; determine the frequency, intensity, and duration of training sessions; choose the level of resistance; and set the pace of progression so that your body's response to strength training will be a series of positive adaptations and not aggravations.

Let us deal with each of these important aspects of strength training and look at how to make our exercising safe.

Exercise Selection

You can choose from a wide range of strength-training exercises with various degrees of difficulty and complexity. If you start strength training after a long period of inactivity and your level of strength fitness is fairly low, *it is wise to select simple and relatively easy exercises for your initial program.* Raise the level of your strength and skills with these simple and less demanding exercises in a patient and gradual manner. *Progress toward more complicated and difficult exercises only after your gains are consolidated and confirmed.*

For example: for beginners with low strength and skill level, it is wise to choose wall push-ups (also called push-aways) initially and leave regular push-ups for later. Exercise your legs by standing up from a bench and postpone squats for when your leg strength and sense of balance improve. Beginners should also avoid overhead movements with weights and exercises that involve countermovements, such as lunges. Generally speaking, always stay within your comfort level and always make sure that the exercises you choose are not straining your body and that you are not overextending your abilities.

Frequency of Workouts

Always remember that *when you work out, the exercises you perform will stress your tissues* and this stress includes microscopic damage to your muscles, tendons, and ligaments. Stressed tissues must undergo a repair and rebuilding process that may last for forty-eight to ninety-six hours. If you give your body the necessary time to repair and rebuild, you will steadily improve in your strength fitness. On the other hand, if you do a workout before the repair and rebuilding processes are completed, your tissues will slowly degrade. However, if you wait too long until the next workout, your body (use it or lose it principle) passes over the optimal period of readiness and you will experience little or no progress.

I find that *two or three training sessions a week on non-consecutive days is the optimal training frequency for strength training.* To make sure that recovery is complete, I like to train the lower body and torso in one session and the upper body and torso in the next. The muscles of the torso—because of the lack of joints, tendons, and ligaments and because of the proximity to large blood vessels—tend to recover faster.

Intensity of Workouts

When it comes to physical training, *intensity is the amount of work done within a certain period.* The more work you compress into a workout, the heavier the resistance you use, the faster your movements are, and the less rest you take between sets and exercises, the more intense your workouts become.

For seniors—especially when they embark on a strength-training program—I recommend that they *keep the intensity of their workouts from low to moderate.* By this I mean exercising against low to moderate resistance, performing the movements slowly, and taking plenty of rest between sets of exercises. The time between sets and various exercises should be used for stretching, breathing, and visualizing (mentally rehearsing) the next exercise or set.

Duration of Workouts

Depending on the health, fitness status, and biological age of the person, the duration of each strength-training session can be anything between twenty to sixty minutes. *It is safer to start with shorter sessions and gradually increase workout time as you progress.*

Resistance

Resistance, be it gravity or an elastic band, *is the opposing force pitted against the force of your muscles in action.* Your muscles may defeat that force, may hold a contraction against it without producing any movement, or may just have to yield to it while trying to resist it. In my opinion, seniors should stay away from holding against a force (by isometric muscle action) and should not work against resistance that would force their muscles to yield (eccentric muscle action). This means that the resistance for strength training is the force we are able to defeat by producing a muscle contraction that will result in the desired movement (concentric muscle action).

What is the best way of determining the optimal resistance (the opposing force) you want to tackle to exercise your muscles? If I say that you should exercise your muscles against a force that is about 75 percent of the maximum force you can produce, I might tempt you to test your maximum strength, and no senior should ever do that. *The best and safest way of determining optimal resistance is to perform a particular exercise and adjust the resistance until you find that you can execute the movement eight to twelve times (eight to twelve repetitions) without straining while maintaining correct form, proper posture, and proper breathing pattern.*

Three sets of eight to twelve repetitions with two or three minutes of rest between each set is a good protocol to achieve optimal strength gains safely and effectively.

Pace of Progression

Progression is the movement in the direction of your goals. When it comes to progression, my most important observation in training myself and in training and observing others is that *rushing progression is hindering it.*

Whenever you increase the rate and pace of progression above what is optimal, you not only risk injuries, plateaus, burnouts, and maladaptations (negative responses), you also upset the body's rhythm and cycle of absorbing stress and repairing and rebuilding by imposing more stress on it through heavier workloads. The result can be physically and psychologically devastating.

It is very important to exercise prudence and patience and plan progression so that *your workouts are challenging, but not aggravating your body.*

At the beginning, improvements are usually quite spectacular. It is quite normal to experience a 50–75 percent increase in your strength during the first couple of months of strength training, but this increase in your ability to perform more work is due mostly to neural rather than anatomical adaptations. This means that although there is very little improvement in the strength of the individual muscles and muscle fibers, you still become able to perform more work because your central nervous system learns how to organize, coordinate, and recruit your individual muscles and muscle fibers more efficiently. This means that the physical resources remain just about the same, but the nervous system, through more efficient processing and more effective control mechanisms, is able to get more work out of your muscles.

It is a mistake to think that this fast initial rate of progress will be a permanent pace of improvement in your physical strength. How do you determine your optimal rate of progression?

Set the initial resistance at a level against which you can perform a particular exercise eight to twelve times. Make sure that the exercise is performed correctly with correct posture and proper breathing. When you are able to perform sixteen repetitions of the same exercise in three sets correctly without overextending and straining yourself, you can firmly establish strength gains for a week, improving all aspects of your form. After this week of consolidation, increase resistance so that you can perform the same exercise only eight to twelve times while maintaining correct form and without straining yourself.

Later in your progress there will be a limit to how much you can increase the level of resistance. It is a common mistake and a source of possible injuries and disappointments to measure improvements solely by the amount (quantity) of work you are able to perform. There are other aspects of improvement that reflect qualitative changes, such as skill levels, postural improvements, and better gait. Because there is a limit to the amount of force you will be able to generate, the simple-minded preoccupation with being able to work against heavier and heavier resistance will limit your prospects. At the same time, there is almost no end to learning and refining skills.

I highly recommend widening the scope of your aspirations and

- perfect your form and technical skills
- increase the variety of exercises
- increase the level of complexity of the exercises

- introduce new training modalities into your program, such as various recreational and competitive activities (canoeing, kayaking, hiking, swimming, etc.)

Various Other Considerations

Although we will deal with the importance of a proper warm-up, cool-down, stretching, and performing exercises in their full range of motion, I will briefly deal with these aspects of safety in this chapter.

A warm-up—that is, the gradual increase in your body's activity level—is a very important way of avoiding injuries. It improves circulation (safely elevating heart rate and expanding the walls of blood vessels), leads to more efficient metabolism (elevating the intensity of transport of nutrients to the working muscles and removal of waste products), increases awareness, refreshes muscle memory, and raises the level of preparedness of your bodily systems so that they will be better able to meet the demands of strength training.

A *cool-down*, on the other hand, by allowing your bodily systems to slowly lower the level of intensity of their operations, *will ensure a smooth transition from an active to less active state* and will help avoid aggravations that might happen if you abruptly stop working out. When exercisers and trainers talk about the importance of a full range of motion, some fail to mention that "full" is a relative term because every individual has a different level of joint mobility. Furthermore, that individual level may change from time to time, from one exercise to the other, and may also vary according to the level of resistance.

You should never force your joints and move beyond a pain-free range of motion. Always stay within your comfort level and avoid straining your joints. Always go to the point of pain, but never through pain.

Effective

An effective program or procedure produces the best possible results consistently. We have already dealt with some aspects of effective training when we discussed the various requirements of safe exercising. Under this heading, we deal only with the ability to produce the best results consistently. This is the ability to bring out the best in your body, to *elicit maximum gains and realize your maximum potential* without losing sight of safety and without stepping over the boundaries of prudence and reason.

An effective program will provide optimal stimulus and challenge for your body. If the level, quality, and nature of the stimuli are just about right at the beginning of your program and is progressively adjusted as your strength fitness improves, you will achieve your maximum potential.

You must consider every aspect of your health and fitness, your biological age, your level of activity, and your goals in order to determine the most effective way of improving your strength fitness. For example, although it might improve your muscle speed and coordination, table tennis is not an effective way of improving your strength fitness, nor is bowling. Physical labor—from low-intensity activities such as gardening to plastering an old wall—is not an effective form of strength training either. Working out with a balance board and an exercise ball are useful exercise modalities together with yoga and breathing exercises, but are not the most effective forms of strength training.

It has been proven that the most effective way of improving your strength fitness is resistance training, but resistance training must meet certain requirements in order to be effective.

If we use a resistance that is too low to stimulate our muscles or if we use the same monotonous routine each time we train, we will not achieve our maximum potential.

In order for the muscles to become as strong as they can be, our strength-training program must be physically and mentally challenging, stimulating, and changing. It must provide the optimal maximum impact on the muscles to which they can respond positively.

Personalized

One of the basic problems with most popular programs is that they may satisfy the general needs of an arbitrary established statistical average, but fail to address the specific needs, goals, and aspirations of the individual.

It is very important that the program we design and execute fit our needs rather than us trying to fit the program. It is always the program that must be designed, reassessed, and adjusted to suit us and not the other way around.

It is always the program that fails the individual. The individual should never feel obliged to adjust his or her goals and aspirations or to override personal and specific health and fitness concerns in order to satisfy the prescriptions of any program.

When a person forces the various systems of his or her body to absorb and adapt to a program that is not designed to meet his or her individual needs, the following physical maladaptations (negative responses) to exercise may occur:

- acute and chronic injuries and illnesses
- muscle imbalance
- lack of gains in strength
- lack of maintainable progress

The psychological effects of a general program that is not designed to meet the specific needs of the individual, and is not constantly adjusted to your changing needs, can be devastating and may result in:

- low self-esteem resulting from a perception that you are not good enough to execute the program
- frustration resulting from lack of positive stimuli and positive response
- generally negative feelings toward exercise, resulting in lack of enjoyment and satisfaction and, finally, in quitting exercising.

It is very important to design your own personalized program by acquainting yourself with the basics of strength training and learning as much as you can about your state of health and fitness. You must also constantly reassess and readjust it to your changing needs. This personalized program, which will evolve by thoughtful planning as much as by trial and error, will fit your specific needs and will move you toward your own goals safely and effectively.

The process of developing a personalized program will be more demanding mentally than simply adopting a general program, but efforts will be rewarded by:

- learning more about yourself, your abilities, and potential during the process
- having the satisfaction of taking responsibility and independent action
- enjoying a sense of empowerment through defining your goals and aspirations
- enjoying active and informed participation in planning, assessing, and shaping your program (even if some of the above is done in consultation with a fitness professional)
- achieving better results

Initially, it is helpful to consult a qualified fitness professional. This investment might save you from frustrations resulting from unproductive and misdirected efforts.

Functional

Your exercise program must be functional, which means that gains in strength must be translated into real-life abilities.

The narrow muscle-by-muscle, exercise-by-exercise interpretation of muscle strength can be misleading. As a result of this interpretation, some exercisers work their muscles in isolation, and completely disregarding the fact that the practical usefulness of muscle strength gained in such a manner is usually quite small. You may improve the ability of the triceps to extend your arm against resistance, and you may also improve the ability of the biceps to flex your arm more powerfully, but if your exercises focus on only one or two muscle groups with very little or no involvement from the rest of your body, the strength you gain will not be functional.

The long-term goal of improving your strength is not to enable you to do more biceps curls, squats, and abdominal curls, but to make sure that you enjoy life through physical independence and the ability to participate in various satisfying physical activities. To gain muscle strength is a good immediate, short-term goal, but the long-term goal is to have strength that improves your quality of life, not just that of your individual muscles.

How do we transform the extra strength your muscles gain into more powerful real-life movement and the ability to participate in real-life activities?

One way is to gradually widen the range of exercises so that they involve more and more muscles. As your overall strength increases, you can also include more difficult and more complex exercises that require the coordinated participation of your whole body. Another way of achieving functional strength is to perform the exercises in ways that resemble real-life demands and situations requiring balance, agility, and various other skills. Instead of performing some exercises on a bench, you can do them on an exercise ball. At a certain point you might want to participate in various recreational or competitive activities that can range from hiking and swimming to playing tennis and canoeing.

Progressive

As we have already mentioned in the section dealing with safety, *progression is the act of moving forward in the direction of your goals.* Depending on your genetics, biological age, health, and fitness status, you have a certain strength potential. The realization of this potential is one of your long-term goals. Using progressive strength-training methods, you will be able to move toward this goal.

Strength has many aspects such as:

- maximum strength, which is measured by the maximum resistance you are able to defeat
- relative strength, which is your strength measured relative to your body weight
- strength endurance, which is your ability to repeatedly defeat resistance for a prolonged period
- functional strength, which is the strength needed to perform real-life tasks

While progression in maximum strength and relative strength is a valid goal and certainly the easiest to measure, I discourage seniors from focusing solely on improving their maximum strength. I strongly recommend that you avoid testing your maximum or relative strength.

In order for you to progress in every aspect of your strength fitness, your program must include the following:

- a progressive and gradual increase in the resistance your muscles must defeat (interspersed with periods of consolidation)
- a progressive increase in the variety of exercises
- a progressive increase in the difficulty and complexity of exercises and activities

Balanced

A balanced strength-training program will ensure that *the whole musculature of your body is improved proportionately.* If we widen the concept of balance to include all aspects of fitness, we mean that every important component of your fitness is properly considered and improved in a balanced manner. You may have a certain bias for a particular aspect of fitness (such as strength), but you should not disregard other important components, such as flexibility.

Designing Your Initial Program

You already know the basic training principles. They will provide you with general guidelines that must be considered in devising any strength-training program. In this chapter I will provide a few practical examples of program design with hypothetical medical and fitness parameters. You will see that whatever your health and fitness status, and whatever your biological age, there is no reason to postpone your program toward increased strength and all the rewards that come with it.

Every conscious act starts in the mind. Let us imagine a few scenarios and put the knowledge base we have built to some practical use and design a few strength-training programs.

Program #1

Let us imagine that you are a typical senior who has been cleared by your doctor for strength training. You have high blood pressure, arthritis in the hips and knees, and you are overweight by about 25 lbs (11 kg). The combined result of arthritis and excess weight make it difficult for you to get up from the sitting position. You have been sedentary for the last ten years. Your chronological age is 60, but the combined effects of bad lifestyle habits, a sedentary life, and medical conditions such as high blood pressure and arthritis puts your biological age closer to 60.

You have already made up your mind to become physically active. You have started working on your lifestyle habits and have made significant changes in the right direction. You have also taken the first step toward being more active by starting to walk and presently walk for 20 minutes a day before dinner.

It would make sense to plan two strength-training sessions per week initially with two or three days between each session. Later when your fitness improves, you might want to increase it to three sessions per week.

It would also make good sense to exercise for 15 to 20 minutes each time. Wait until your body consistently responds well to strength training for a month before you gradually increase the duration of each strength-training session.

Because of your high blood pressure, the length of inactivity, and the resulting biological age, you should start your strength training with very simple exercises. You should also avoid the risks of high blood pressure by including only those exercises that are performed in the upright position, such as wall quarter squats performed against minimal resistance. (For wall quarter squats, lean against a wall and, with legs shoulder-width apart, flex your knees about 25°, then extend your legs. When the combined effects of good lifestyle habits and walking lower your weight and blood pressure, you can then include exercises that require other than an upright position.

Both your legs and upper body are relatively weak. Your arthritis and the extra weight you carry make every exercise more difficult to perform.

Considering all the above, it is reasonable to suggest that initially, you should do only two exercises for the legs, three exercises for the upper body, and one for your abs.

Start with a warm-up. Walk in place for a few minutes while maintaining correct posture and doing deep inhales and full exhales.

For your legs, you should do three sets of eight to twelve wall quarter squats, rest for about two minutes between each set by walking in place, and do deep inhales and full exhales.

The next leg exercise is leg abductions, which you perform while standing and facing a wall. Lean against it with arms in the push-up position and slowly and continuously raise one of your legs laterally (sideways), then lower the leg just as slowly. Do three sets of eight to twelve repetitions for each leg with two minutes of active rest between sets. Active rest may be walking in place while practising deep inhales and full exhales.

At the beginning you will find that it is difficult to raise your leg more than 15°–20°. You should not force your range of motion beyond what you are comfortable with.

With high blood pressure, you should not do abdominal crunches while lying on the floor, at least not until the combined effects of good lifestyle habits, walking, strength training, and breathing lower your blood pressure.

The safest abdominal exercise for your health and fitness status is to sit on a chair or a bench and slowly raise one bent knee toward your chest while you exhale, hold the knee raised for a moment, then lower it slowly as you inhale. Repeat the exercise eight to twelve times for each leg, stand up between sets, walk in place, and perform deep inhales and full exhales. In a few weeks you may want to sit on a chair placed far enough away from a table so that you can reach the tabletop comfortably with your hands to support yourself and raise both bent knees slowly toward your chest.

For a cool-down, repeat your warm-up of walking in place while maintaining correct posture and breathing with deep inhales and full exhales.

In a few weeks, as your legs get stronger, you can add exercises such as heel raises to this lower-body/torso routine. You can also switch from quarter to half squats.

For upper body exercises you can do wall push-ups and biceps curls at the beginning. Later, as your fitness improves, you can add other exercises such as lateral arm raises.

Do your usual warm-up of walking in place and practising deep inhales and full exhales. Stand facing a wall, just far enough away that your extended arms can reach the wall at shoulder height and a little wider than shoulder width. Lean against the wall by slightly bending your elbows. Exhale. Inhale as you bend your elbows and lean toward the wall. Bend your elbows as much as you feel comfortable with. Stop. Slowly push yourself away from the wall as you exhale. Perform eight to twelve repetitions in three sets with active rest between sets.

The next exercise is biceps curls, which you can do standing or standing with your back against a wall.

With one 2.5–5 lb (1–2 kg) dumbbell in each hand, stand with your feet shoulder-width apart. Exhale. Inhale as you slowly raise the dumbbells to the level of your shoulders while keeping the elbows against your side. Lower the dumbbells slowly as you exhale. Repeat eight to twelve times and have two minutes of active rest, which can be rotating your shoulders back and forth with your arms hanging by your side and practising deep inhales and full exhales. Do three sets of biceps curls, then continue with your next exercise.

Your next exercise is lateral arm raises. Stand with your feet a little wider than shoulder width. Do a few deep inhales and full exhales. Exhale as you laterally raise your arms up to shoulder height, hold your arms in the horizontal position for a moment, and inhale as you slowly lower them. Repeat this exercise eight to twelve times and have two minutes of active rest, which can be rotating your shoulder back and forth and practising deep inhales and full exhales. Later, as your deltoid muscles become stronger, you can perform this exercise with a 1.5 lb (0.5 kg) dumbbell.

Continue with your abdominal exercises, which will be the same as the ones you did after your leg exercise routine.

End your session with five minutes of cool-down, consisting of walking in place while maintaining good posture. Repeat the biceps curls without weights a few times and practise deep inhales and full exhales.

In a few weeks as your upper body gets stronger, you can add an exercise such as one-arm rowing (initially, use a 5–10 lb/2–4.5 kg) dumbbell) to this upper-body/torso routine.

See the exercise sheets (lower body/torso and upper body/torso) for Program #1 for beginners with low fitness level and a medical condition such as high blood pressure.

NOTE: *You will find blank exercise sheets for lower body/torso, upper body/torso and stability ball exercises at the end of the book. You can copy them and use them to design your own exercise programs.*

NB: Copy this sheet and file with your fitness documents		Date:	Date:	Date:	Date:	Date:	Date:	Date:
Exercise:	RESIST:	Self	Self	Self				
quarter	1st set	12	14	16				
squats	2nd set	12	14	16				
	3rd set	12	14	16				
Exercise:	RESIST:				Self	Self	Self	Self
half	1st set				12	14	16	16
squats	2nd set				12	14	16	16
	3rd set				12	14	16	16
Exercise:	RESIST:	Self	Self	Self	Self	Self	Self	Self
leg	1st set	12	14	16	16	16	16	16
abductions	2nd set	12	14	16	16	16	16	16
	3rd set	12	14	16	16	16	16	16
Exercise:	RESIST:			Self	Self	Self	Self	Self
heel	1st set			12	14	16	16	16
raises	2nd set			12	14	16	16	16
	3rd set			12	14	16	16	16
Exercise:	RESIST:							
	1st set							
	2nd set							
	3rd set							
Exercise:	RESIST:	Self	Self	Self				
abs:	1st set	12	14	16				
alternate	2nd set	12	14	16				
knee raises	3rd set	12	14	16				
Exercise:	RESIST:				Self	Self	Self	Self
simultaneous	1st set				12	12	12	14
knee raises	2nd set				12	12	12	14
	3rd set				12	12	12	14

Program #1   Upper Body/Torso

Exercise:	RESIST:	Date:	Date:	Date:	Date:	Date:	Date:	Date:
wall push-ups	RESIST:	Self	Self	Self	Self	Self	Self	Self
	1st set	8	12	14	16	16	16	16
	2nd set	8	10	12	14	16	16	16
	3rd set	8	10	12	14	16	16	16
Exercise: biceps curls	RESIST:	5 lbs (2 kg)	5 lbs (2 kg)	5 lbs (2 kg)	5 lbs (2 kg)	8 lbs (3.5 kg)	8 lbs (3.5 kg)	8 lbs (3.5 kg)
	1st set	8	10	12	12	8	10	12
	2nd set	8	10	12	12	8	10	12
	3rd set	8	10	12	12	8	10	12
Exercise: lateral arm raises	RESIST:			Self	Self	Self	1.5 lbs (.5 kg)	1.5 lbs (.5 kg)
	1st set			8	10	12	8	10
	2nd set			8	10	12	8	10
	3rd set			8	10	12	8	10
Exercise:	RESIST:							
	1st set							
	2nd set							
	3rd set							
Exercise: abs: alternate knee raises	RESIST:	Self	Self	Self				
	1st set	12	14	16				
	2nd set	12	14	16				
	3rd set	12	14	16				
Exercise: simultaneous knee raises	RESIST:				Self	Self	Self	Self
	1st set				12	14	16	16
	2nd set				12	14	16	16
	3rd set				12	14	16	16
Exercise:	RESIST:							
	1st set							
	2nd set							
	3rd set							

Program #2

Let's assume you have no medical problems and that your doctor has cleared you for strength training. You are active and walk daily for about 45 minutes. You do gardening from spring to late fall and spend winters in the south where, besides your daily walk, you swim and occasionally play golf. Your lifestyle habits are good except for problems related to managing stress, but you recognized the symptoms, identified the sources, and are well on your way to developing your coping skills. Your chronological age is 80, but your biological age—thanks to the regular physical activities, good nutrition, and steadily improving ability to cope with stress—is in the mid-70s. You have noticed some loss of muscle and decrease in strength and want to embark on a strength-training program. You went to your local YMCA for a fitness assessment. Your strength is average for your age, but your posture needs improvement. You have the tendency to hunch your back and to let your shoulders fall forward. The fitness professional doing the assessment recommended that you work on your middle trapezoids, rhomboids, your scapular stabilizers, and spinal erectors to correct this problem.

The initial goal of your strength-training program is to strengthen the muscles that keep your spine in correct, neutral position and stop your shoulders from hunching.

The safest and most effective way to strengthen these muscles is to exercise with a stability ball. These exercises should be done daily. (Stability ball exercises will be described in detail in the next chapter.)

The three exercises that you should do daily to strengthen the middle trapezoids, rhomboids, scapular stabilizers, and spinal erectors are the following:

Position yourself on the exercise ball so that your chest and stomach are on the ball and your hands and knees are on the floor. Slowly lift the opposite arm and leg, pause, and lower them just as slowly. Inhale as you lift the opposite arm and leg and exhale as you lower them. Repeat, lifting the other opposite arm and leg. Do eight to twelve repetitions in three sets and rock on the ball back and forth, relaxed between each set. (See stability ball exercises.)

With the ball under your chest and stomach, slowly walk forward so that the ball will roll back and will be under your pelvis. Walk backwards just as slowly and with small steps. Repeat this exercise six to eight times in three sets and rock on the ball back and forth, relaxed between each set. (See stability ball exercises.)

Assume the same position on the exercise ball. The ball sits under your chest and stomach, and your knees and hands are on the floor. Press your stomach and pelvis into the ball. Lift your chest and raise your elbows behind your back. Hold this position for a moment, then go back to the original prone position on the ball as you exhale. Repeat this exercise eight to twelve times and relax on the ball, rocking back and forth between each set. (See stability ball exercises.)

You can start with one session of lower-body/torso and one session of upper-body/torso exercises per week done on non-consecutive days.

Because you are fairly fit, the duration of each session can be 30 to 45 minutes at the beginning and increased to 60 minutes in a few months by adding additional exercises to both your lower-body/torso and upper-body/torso routine.

See the exercise sheets on the following page for Program #2 and the description of exercises in Chapter 7.

NOTE: *You will find blank exercise sheets for lower-body/torso, upper-body/torso, and stability ball exercises at the end of the book.*

For seniors who have been inactive for most of their adult lives, have poor balance, are obese and lack sufficient musle strength to perform the exercises in these initial programs designed for a typical elderly person, should start with a series of beginner exercises:

Program #2   Stability Ball Exercises

NB: Copy this sheet and file with your fitness documents		Date:	Date:	Date:	Date:	Date:	Date:	Date:
Exercise:	RESIST:	Self	Self	Self	Self	Self	Self	Self
lifting	1st set	8	10	12	14	16	16	16
opposite arms	2nd set	8	10	12	14	16	16	16
and legs	3rd set	8	10	12	14	16	16	16
Exercise:	RESIST:	Self	Self	Self	Self	Self	Self	Self
walk	1st set	6	8	10	12	14	16	16
out and back	2nd set	6	8	10	12	14	16	16
	3rd set	6	8	10	12	14	16	16
Exercise:	RESIST:	Self	Self	Self	Self	Self	Self	Self
back	1st set	8	10	12	14	16	16	16
extension or	2nd set	8	10	12	14	16	16	16
curl back	3rd set	8	10	12	14	16	16	16
Exercise:	RESIST:							
	1st set							
	2nd set							
	3rd set							
Exercise:	RESIST:							
	1st set							
	2nd set							
	3rd set							
Exercise:	RESIST:							
	1st set							
	2nd set							
	3rd set							
Exercise:	RESIST:							
	1st set							
	2nd set							
	3rd set							

Program #2   Lower Body/Torso

NB: Copy this sheet and file with your fitness documents

Exercise:	RESIST:	Date: 10 lbs (4.5 kg)	Date: 10 lbs (4.5 kg)	Date: 10 lbs (4.5 kg)	Date: 12 lbs (5.5 kg)	Date: 12 lbs (5.5 kg)	Date: 12 lbs (5.5 kg)	Date: 15 lbs (7 kg)
dumbbell squats	1st set	8	10	12	8	10	12	8
	2nd set	8	10	12	8	10	12	8
	3rd set	8	10	12	8	10	12	8
Exercise: lateral leg raises	RESIST:	Self	Self	Self	Self	Self	Self	Self
	1st set	8 per leg	10 per leg	12 per leg	14 per leg	16 per leg	16 per leg	16 per leg
	2nd set	8 per leg	10 per leg	12 per leg	14 per leg	16 per leg	16 per leg	16 per leg
	3rd set	8 per leg	10 per leg	12 per leg	14 per leg	16 per leg	16 per leg	16 per leg
Exercise: forward lunges	RESIST:	Self	Self	Self	Self	Self	Self	Self
	1st set	8 per leg	10 per leg	12 per leg	14 per leg	16 per leg	16 per leg	16 per leg
	2nd set	8 per leg	10 per leg	12 per leg	14 per leg	16 per leg	16 per leg	16 per leg
	3rd set	8 per leg	10 per leg	12 per leg	14 per leg	16 per leg	16 per leg	16 per leg
Exercise: heel raises	RESIST:	Self	Self	Self	Self	Self	Self	Self
	1st set	8	10	12	14	16	16	16
	2nd set	8	10	12	14	16	16	16
	3rd set	8	10	12	14	16	16	16
Exercise: leg adductions (Stability Ball)	RESIST:	Ball	Ball	Ball	Ball	Ball	Ball	Ball
	1st set	8	10	12	14	16	16	16
	2nd set	8	10	12	14	16	16	16
	3rd set	8	10	12	14	16	16	16
Exercise: trunk curls	RESIST:	Self	Self	Self	Self	Self	Self	Self
	1st set	8	10	12	14	16	16	16
	2nd set	8	10	12	14	16	16	16
	3rd set	8	10	12	14	16	16	16
Exercise: back extension (Stability Ball)	RESIST:	Self	Self	Self	Self	Self	Self	Self
	1st set	8	10	12	14	16	16	16
	2nd set	8	10	12	14	16	16	16
	3rd set	8	10	12	14	16	16	16

Program #2   Upper Body/Torso

NB: Copy this sheet and file with your fitness documents		Date:	Date:	Date:	Date:	Date:	Date:	Date:
Exercise:	RESIST:	12 lbs (5.5 kg)	12 lbs (5.5 kg)	12 lbs (5.5 kg)	12 lbs (5.5 kg)	15 lbs (7 kg)	15 lbs (7 kg)	15 lbs (7 kg)
dumbbell chest press	1st set	8	10	12	12	8	10	12
	2nd set	8	10	12	12	8	10	12
	3rd set	8	10	12	12	8	10	12
Exercise:	RESIST:	12 lbs (5.5 kg)	12 lbs (5.5 kg)	12 lbs (5.5 kg)	12 lbs (5.5 kg)	15 lbs (5.5 kg)	15 lbs (5.5 kg)	15 lbs (5.5 kg)
one-arm rowing	1st set	8	10	12	12	8	10	12
	2nd set	8	10	12	12	8	10	12
	3rd set	8	10	12	12	8	10	12
Exercise:	RESIST:	10 lbs (4.5 kg)	10 lbs (4.5 kg)	10 lbs (4.5 kg)	12 lbs (5.5 kg)	12 lbs (5.5 kg)	12 lbs (5.5 kg)	12 lbs (5.5 kg)
biceps curls	1st set	8	10	12	12	8	10	12
	2nd set	8	10	12	12	8	10	12
	3rd set	8	10	12	12	8	10	12
Exercise:	RESIST:	15 lbs (7 kg)	15 lbs (7 kg)	15 lbs (7 kg)	15 lbs (7 kg)	20 lbs (9 kg)	20 lbs (9 kg)	20 lbs (9 kg)
chest pullover	1st set	8	10	12	12	8	10	12
	2nd set	8	10	12	12	8	10	12
	3rd set	8	10	12	12	8	10	12
Exercise:	RESIST:	8 lbs (3.5 kg)	8 lbs (3.5 kg)	8 lbs (3.5 kg)	8 lbs (3.5 kg)	10 lbs (4.5 kg)	10 lbs (4.5 kg)	10 lbs (4.5 kg)
lateral arm raises	1st set	8	10	12	12	8	10	12
	2nd set	8	10	12	12	8	10	12
	3rd set	8	10	12	12	8	10	12
Exercise:	RESIST:	Self	Self	Self	Self	Self	Self	Self
trunk curls	1st set	10	12	14	16	16	16	16
	2nd set	10	12	14	16	16	16	16
	3rd set	10	12	14	16	16	16	16
Exercise:	RESIST:	Self	Self	Self	Self	Self	Self	Self
trunk cross curls	1st set	6	8	10	12	14	16	16
	2nd set	6	8	10	12	14	16	16
	3rd set	6	8	10	12	14	16	16

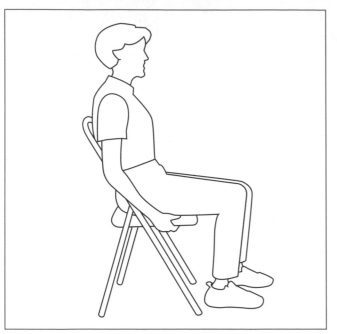

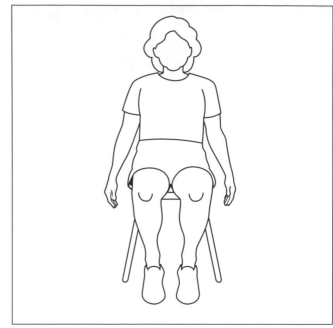

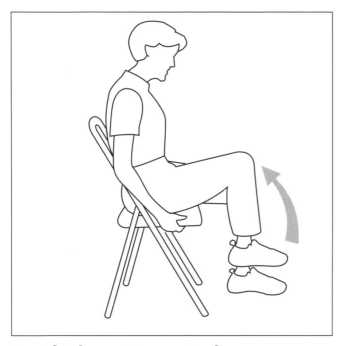

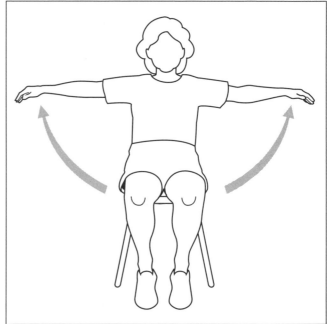

1. Sitting Knee Raise

Muscles participating:
iliopsoas, abdominals
- Sit on a chair.
- Raise one bent knee toward your chest.
- Then lower knee.
- Repeat with the other knee.

2. Sitting Arm Abduction

Muscles participating:
Deltoids and upper trapezoids
- Sit on a chair with your arms hanging by your sides.
- Raise arms to horizontal position.

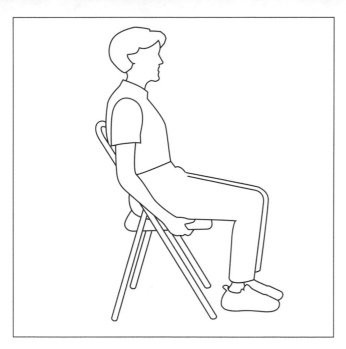

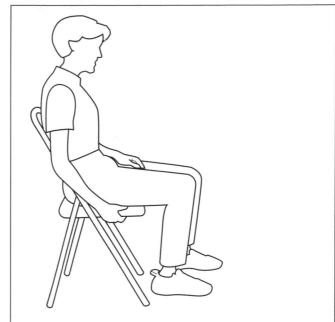

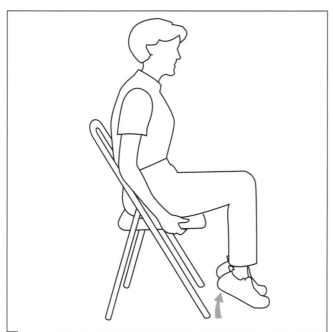

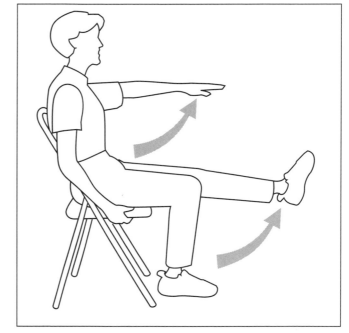

3. Sitting Heel Raise

Muscles participating:
Calves

- Sit on a chair with both feet flat on the floor.
- Slowly raise both heels in a controlled manner.

4. Sitting Arm and Leg Raise

Muscles participating:
Deltoids, quadriceps, and iliopsoas

- Sit on a chair.
- Raise arm and leg on one side simultaneously.
- Repeat with the other side.

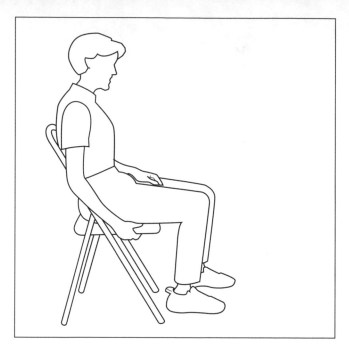

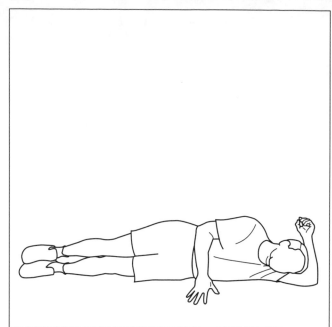

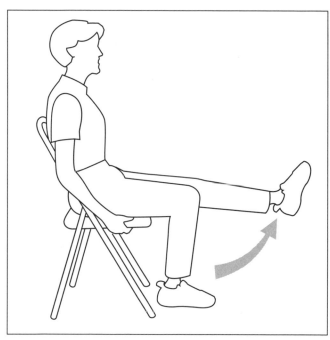

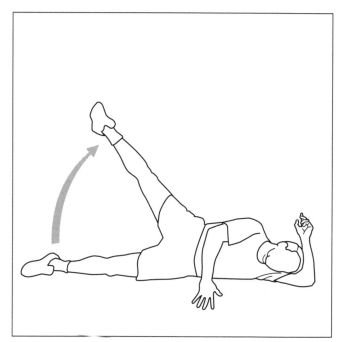

5. Sitting Leg Raise

Muscles participating:

Quadriceps and iliopsoas

- Sit on a chair.
- Slowly raise one leg in a controlled motion and extend it fully as you raise it.
- Lower it slowly.
- Repeat with the other leg.

6. Leg Abduction

Muscles participating:

Gluteus medius and minimus

- Lie on your side with one leg over the other, and one arm under your head. Your other arm is flexed and the hand is flat on the floor.
- Slowly raise the top leg in a controlled motion as high as you can.
- Hold for a moment.
- Lower the leg slowly.

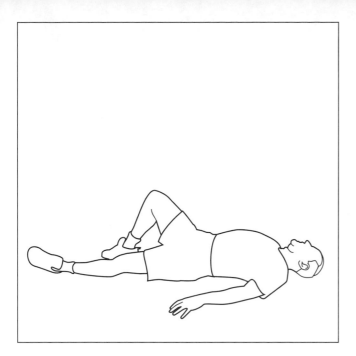

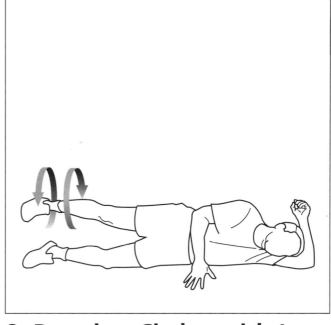

8. Drawing Circles with Leg

Muscles participating:
Gluteus medius and minimus

- Lie on your side with one arm under your head and the other arm flexed over your chest and the hand on the floor.
- Lift leg and draw circles clockwise, then counterclockwise in the air.
- Repeat for the other side.

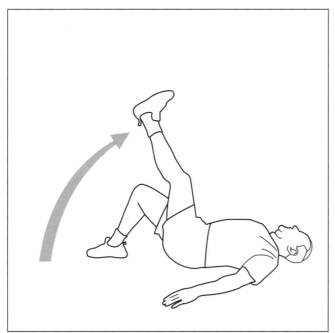

7. Leg Raise

Muscles participating:
iliopsoas, quadriceps, abdominals

- Lie on the floor on your back with one leg extended and the other leg bent.
- Slowly raise the extended leg in a controlled motion.
- Lower leg.

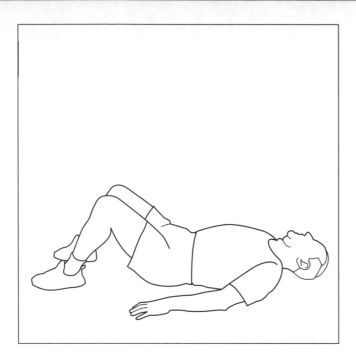

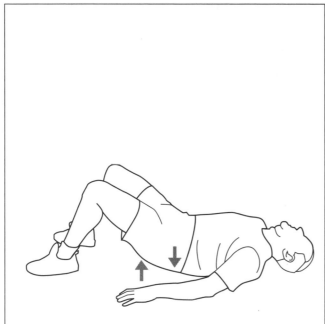

9. Pelvic Tilt

Muscles participating:
Abdominals, iliopsoas

- Lie on your back with your knees bent and your feet flat on the floor.
- Press the small of your back into the floor, contract abdominals, and tilt pelvis upward.
- Lower the pelvis and relax the abdominals.

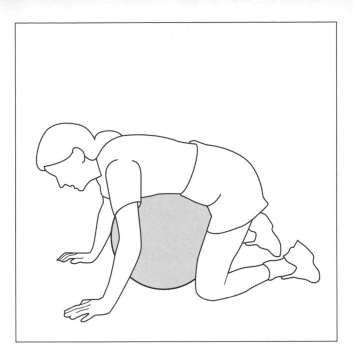

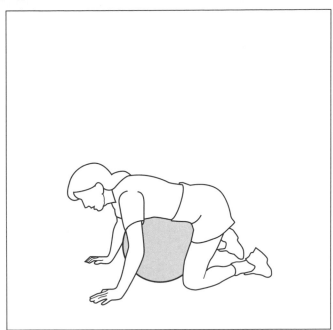

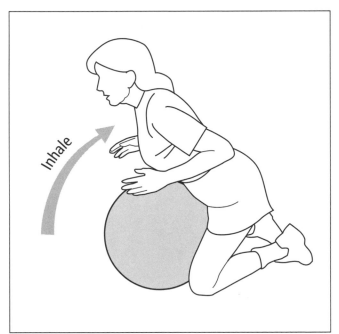

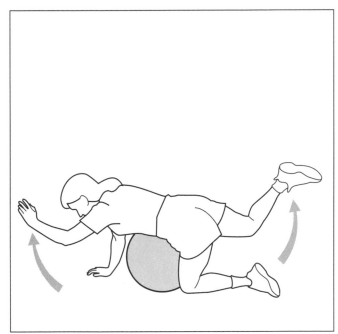

1. Curl Back

Muscles participating:

quadratus lumborum spinal erectors, rhomboids, middle trapezoids

- Crouch over the ball and position it between your knees.
- Press your pelvis into the ball and slowly raise your elbows above your back.
- Maintain this position for a moment, then slowly return to the starting position as you exhale.

2. Lifting Opposite Arm and Leg

Muscles participating:

Scapular stabilizers, rotator cuff, hip extensors

- Position yourself over the ball and exhale.
- Press your abdomen and pelvis into the ball.
- Slowly and simultaneously raise one arm and the opposite leg while inhaling.
- Hold for a moment, lower, and exhale. Repeat the same movement by lifting the other arm and leg.

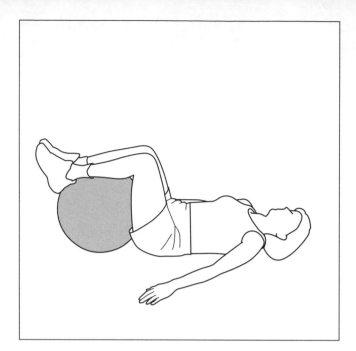

3. Hip Extension

Muscles participating:

Gluteals, quadratus lumborum, spinal erectors

- Lie on your back with legs resting on the ball.
- Inhale.
- Extend your hip by pressing your legs down on the ball and raising your buttocks off the floor.
- Exhale.
- When the hip is extended and buttocks raised, move your hip slowly to the right and then to the left. Breathe regularly.
- Repeat this sideways motion four to six times.
- Lower your buttocks.

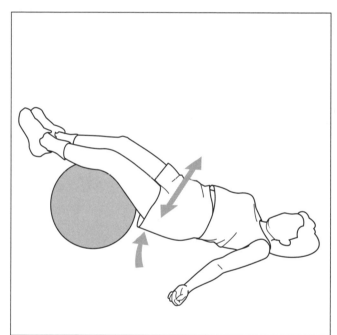

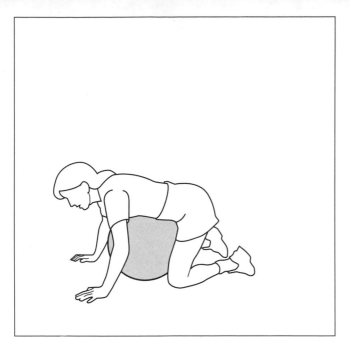

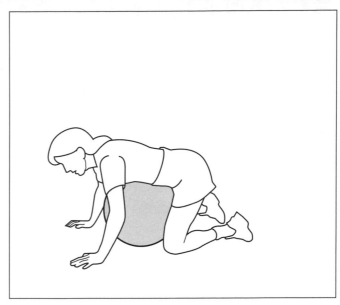

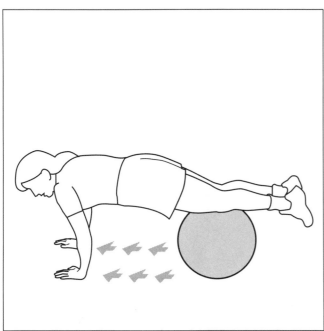

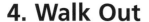

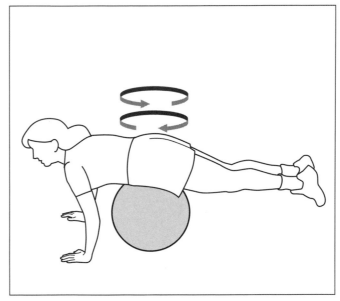

4. Walk Out

Muscles participating:

Rotator cuff, scapular stabilizers, triceps, abdominals.

- Position yourself over the ball, with knees behind the ball.
- Using your arms, slowly propel yourself forward with the ball under your trunk and your legs raised.
- Slowly propel yourself backward.

5. Pelvic Clock

Muscles participating:

Scapular stabilizers, rotator cuff, deltoids, triceps, abdominals, pectorals, abdominals, quadratus lumborum.

- Position yourself on the ball with your knees behind the ball.
- Your hands should be flat on the floor, slightly wider than shoulder width. Using your arms, slowly propel yourself forward until the ball is under your pelvis. Your legs are raised.
- Draw small clockwise circles with your pelvis on the ball, then counterclockwise. Use your arms and shoulders to assist with this movement.
- Slowly propel yourself backward.

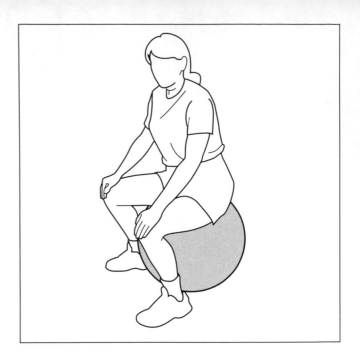

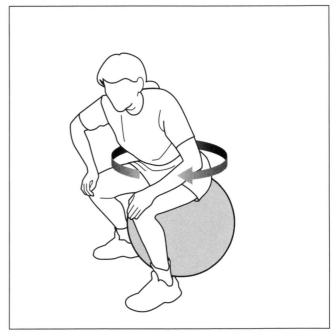

6. Pelvic Circles

Muscles participating:

Abdominals, quadratus lumborum, spinal erectors

- Sit on the ball with your feet flat on the floor, wider than shoulder width apart.
- Rotate your pelvis clockwise a few times, then counterclockwise.

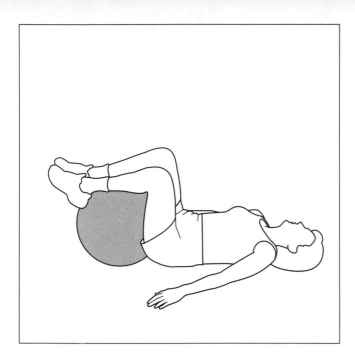

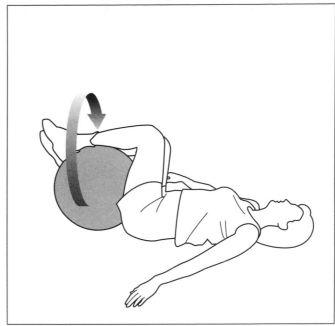

- Bring the ball back to the original position.
- Relax squeeze.

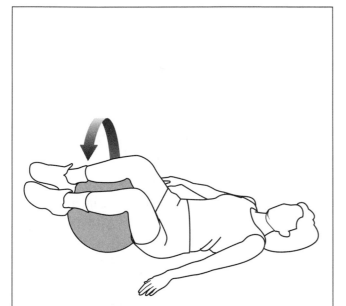

7. Bent-Knee Twist

Muscles participating:

Anterior and posterior obliques, hamstrings

- Place legs on the ball and gently squeeze the ball against your butt.
- Squeeze the ball hard and twist your trunk to the left while lowering your knees to the left.
- Bring the ball back to the original position.
- Relax squeeze.
- Repeat by twisting your trunk to the right while lowering your knees to the right.

It is very important to do your strength-training sessions according to a proper and well-established procedure. To be successful at any endeavor, we need an effective working method—a systematic procedure of getting results.[1] Each exercise has its own special pattern of correct execution. This will be dealt with in a chapter dedicated to the description of various exercises. Regardless of the exercises in each session, each of your training sessions must follow general guidelines that include:

- preparations for a safe training environment
- physical and mental/emotional warm-up
- establishing and maintaining proper posture
- executing movements slowly and in a controlled manner aiming at a full range of motion
- establishing and maintaining a breathing pattern of regular, deep inhales and full exhales
- generating positive feelings related to movements
- performing exercises in a specific order
- cool-down
- stretching

Let us deal with each of these guidelines.

Preparations for a Safe Training Environment

To ensure that accidents will not happen, you must *make sure that your immediate surroundings are safe before each training session:*

- the floor is free of objects that may cause you to trip
- there are no obstructions within your range that would interfere with your movements
- pieces of equipment are orderly, stacked and secured
- equipment, training attire, and shoes are safe and in good working order

Everything—from your shoes and shoelaces to the plates on your dumbbell—must be checked to make sure that accidents do not happen. You might have a safe and effective training program and know how to perform the exercises well, but you can still risk injuries through neglect and lack of care. A plate not secured properly may drop or you can trip over a dumbbell left on the floor. The resulting injuries may set you back for months. A routine visual and manual check of the training area and equipment before each training session will substantially reduce your risk of injuries and will make sure that silly and annoying accidents through neglect and lack of care will not happen.

1. M. Fekete, "The Role of Continuing Education in the NSCA," *Strength and Conditioning* 21, no. 4 (1999): 67–70.

PHYSICAL AND MENTAL/EMOTIONAL WARM-UP

It is very important that you physically and mentally warm up before performing the exercises.

Physical warm-up is absolutely necessary to make sure that your body will react to exercising positively. Any sudden effort may strain your heart and could adversely affect every system from your arteries to your joints and from your muscles to your central nervous system.

While at rest, the various systems of your body are operating at a relatively low level of intensity and readiness. Your heart is beating at a resting heart rate and the diameter of your arteries is calibrated for a normal flow of blood. The release of various enzymes and hormones is slow or at rest. Your joints are not lubricated and your metabolism, including transport of nutrients, and processing and removal of waste products, is idling at best. Your senses are not tuned and the resulting perception may not be as sharp as it should be.

As we age, warm-up becomes even more important because the walls of our arteries are stiffer and need more time to expand for an increased volume of blood. Our joints are dehydrated and need longer to be lubricated by synovial fluid. Our senses and reflexes are slower and need some practice to be alert and to respond promptly.

Do a gentle warm-up by:

* performing rhythmical movements such as walking on a treadmill or walking in place; make sure that your posture is correct, your gait is youthful, and your breathing is efficient

1. Walking in place with knees and elbow drive

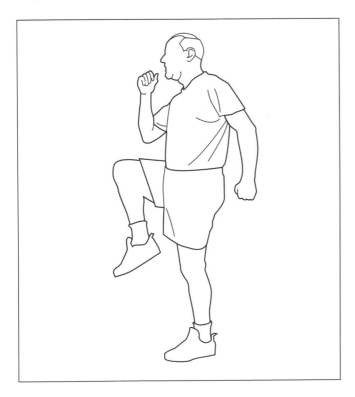
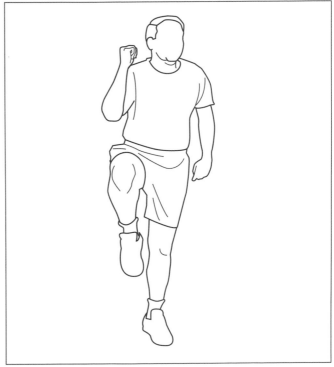

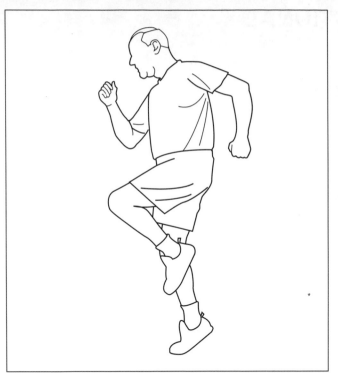

2. Walking on the balls of your feet

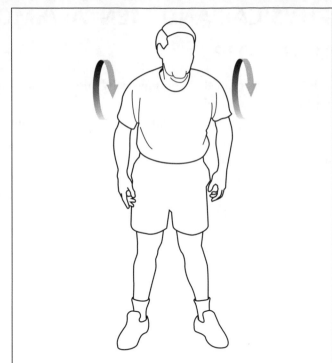

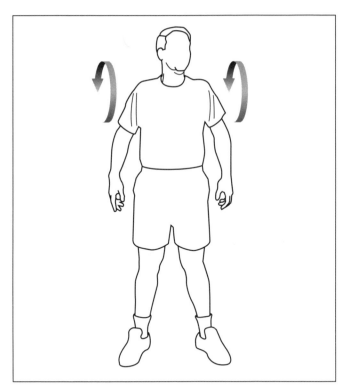

3. Moving your shoulders forward and backward

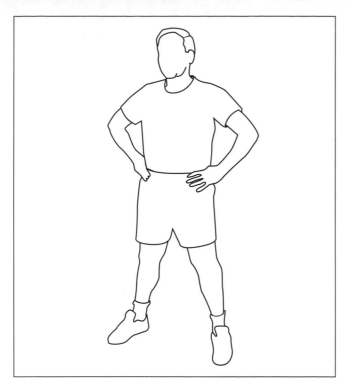

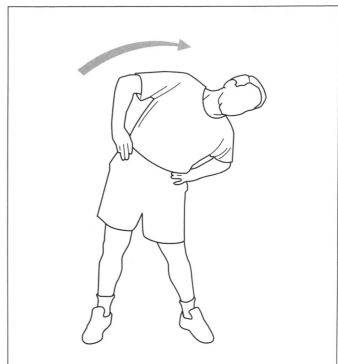

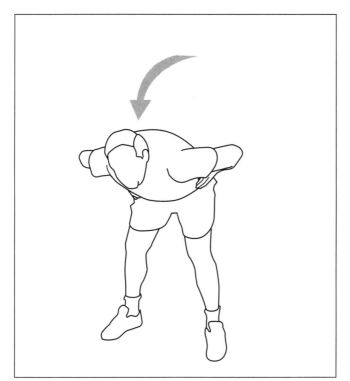

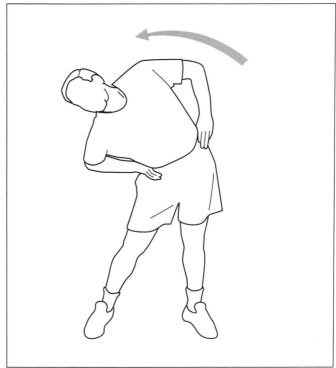

4. Standing good morning

5. Tilting the trunk toward the left, then right

- executing slow, coordinated movements, concentrating on coordination and precision; tense and relax your muscles rhythmically
- doing breathing exercises, focusing on deep inhales and full exhales

After this general physical warm-up, it is recommended, before each exercise, to perform the movements of that particular exercise without resistance a few times. The purpose of this specific warm-up is to practise correct form, correct posture, and correct breathing. It will also refresh muscle memory as it activates the prime movers that will execute the same exercise against resistance.

It is also recommended to go through a mental/emotional rehearsal. *Establishing a positive mindset* at the beginning of each session and maintaining it throughout the whole session *is just as important as a physical warm-up.*

Look forward to each session by generating positive feelings:

- Imagine yourself moving with energy and confidence.
- Visualize yourself performing the exercises with fluid, coordinated, and precise motions.
- Instigate positive emotions by thinking of your session as an important step in your progress toward your goals.

Maintaining Proper Posture

Correct posture is one of the most important aspects of your physical fitness. Together with strength, it also improves your mental/emotional well-being. Although each exercise has its own postural correctness, there are general guidelines that regulate the way we stand and carry ourselves.

At the beginning of each session we must adjust and align the various parts of our bodies by going through the following steps:

- Establish and maintain a correct, neutral alignment of your spine and avoid hunching your back, pushing your head forward, and letting your chin sink toward your chest.
- Once you stand erect, draw your shoulders further back and raise your chest.
- Draw in your stomach further.
- Maintain this healthy posture throughout the session during and between exercises.

At the beginning, it will take constant reminding and constant effort to maintain proper posture, but as you get accustomed to the physical comfort and the better feelings associated with maintaining correct posture, postural awareness and correctness will become automatic.

Movement Speed

It is important to perform the exercises slowly and in a controlled manner. There are several reasons for slow and continuous movements.

If you move too fast, the distribution of work through the range of movement becomes uneven. You preload (overload) the muscles at the beginning of the motion to create speed and the resulting momentum will almost carry the movement through the remaining part of the exercise without requiring much effort from your muscles. With slow and controlled movements, you will distribute force production evenly among the various motor units of your individual muscles through the entire range of motion.

Fast movements will inevitably lead to abrupt rebounding from one to the other end of motion, resulting in sudden countermovements that may strain your joints, tendons, and ligaments. Slow and controlled motions are more forgiving for your joints, tendons, and ligaments.

We will deal with the proper breathing pattern in detail later. When it comes to movement speed, you can use your breathing pattern to set the pace of your movements. Follow the rhythm of deep inhales and full exhales to regulate movement speed. If you make sure that you lower the weight in synch with your full inhale and raise it in tandem with your full exhale, you cannot go wrong with movement speed.

Range of Motion

In strength training it is important to perform exercises in their full range of movement. There are two reasons why we should make it our goal to have a full muscle stretch at the starting position and a full muscle contraction at completion of the movement:

• to develop a full-range of muscle strength at every angle of the motion
• to develop full joint flexibility

However, you must keep in mind that developing full range of movement is a long-term goal, especially for exercisers who have various conditions that restrict range of movement or who start strength training after a long period of inactivity. Biological age also contributes to muscle and joint stiffness.

It is very important that while your goal is to achieve a full range of motion, you should never move beyond a pain-free range of motion. By forcing your joints, muscles, tendons, and ligaments to do something that they are not capable of will inevitably lead to injuries.

If necessary, you must also eliminate exercises that cause immediate or delayed pain at joints. Steady and consistent exercising and keeping movements within a safe and comfortable range will gradually extend your range of motion.

Breathing Pattern

Although I will give specific breathing instructions for each exercise in the book, there are a few general rules that must be followed regardless of the particular exercise.

Do not hold your breath while exercising. You must breathe continuously throughout each repetition of every exercise. Holding your breath while making an effort may produce excessive internal pressure that, in turn, may restrict the flow of blood through your veins back to your heart. This restricted blood flow may cause venous pooling of blood and high blood pressure, and you may experience symptoms such as sudden dizziness and light-headedness that may result in temporary loss of control.

Regulate your breathing. Random breathing, done out of synch with the rhythm of movements, can be just as bad as holding your breath. Fast breathing may cause hyperventilation, may be distracting, and may reduce your ability to exercise control over technique and form. The general rule for regulating breathing is that you exhale when you overcome the resistance (positive phase), and inhale when you yield to resistance (negative phase) to let the contracted muscles stretch and get ready for the next positive phase.

Let us say, for example, that you are performing a wall push-up. Inhale when you move toward the wall and exhale when you push away from the wall.

There are a few exceptions to this general rule. Some fitness books or some trainers recommend that you inhale through the positive phase of the biceps curl and one-arm rowing.

During these exercises, the positive effort is made during the movement toward (rather than away from) the body. While performing both the biceps curl and the one-arm rowing, you defeat resistance when you pull. The expanded chest resulting from the full inhale during the pulling provides a solid platform and ensures correct posture for the exercise.

You can practise one and then the other pattern of breathing while performing these exercises and see which pattern is more suitable for you. If you think that this will be confusing, stick to the general rule of exhaling through the positive phase (overcoming the resistance) and inhaling through the negative phase (yielding to the resistance).

Always inhale fully and exhale fully. It is important that you inhale and exhale fully and slowly in synch with the two movement phases of each exercise. Shallow inhales and exhales will not provide sufficient oxygen for your lungs, reduces the calming effect of slow and deep breathing, and breaks up the rhythm of movement as well as the synch of movement and breathing.

Feeling and Sensations Related to Exercise

In addition to focusing on the exercise, *it is important to generate positive feelings and sensations as you exercise.* Without these positive feelings, exercising would be a chore or a duty and you would act like a robot. In fact, it would be an added stress. Together, intellectual awareness and positive feelings and sensations will mutually enhance each other and will make exercising a satisfying experience.

Positive feelings and sensations act as the driving force behind the knowledge that exercise is good for you. They will add enjoyment to each movement and to each inhale and exhale. These emotions help release endorphins into the bloodstream that, in turn, will further increase the joy and pleasure of exercise. You can double the value of each session by instigating and maintaining positive emotions while exercising.

Here are a few practical tips:

- Enjoy the rhythm of breathing and movement. Be proud of your ability to find your own rhythm.
- Enjoy the good effort you are making. Whenever you sense the negative feeling of resistance bearing down on your muscles, turn it around immediately and feel the force of your muscles defeating that resistance. Enjoy this satisfying feeling.
- Visualize and feel your lungs expanding as you inhale fresh air, and feel the good work your heart does in pumping fresh blood to the working muscles, the lungs, etc.
- In general, feel that you are in your element when you are exercising.

The Order of Exercises

After your usual warm-up, start with exercises that involve the larger muscle groups and leave the smallest muscles for last.

For balanced muscle development, pair exercises, whenever it is possible, so that opposing muscle groups are exercised in direct sequence. For example, after exercising the chest muscles, you should exercise the muscles of the upper back. After exercising the triceps, exercise the biceps, etc. There are exercises that simultaneously exercise the opposing muscle groups, such as the squat, which exercises both the quadriceps and the hamstrings.

Cool-down

A sudden and abrupt cessation of exercising may strain the heart. It is highly recommended that after your regular exercises, you perform certain rhythmical movements, such as walking in place, while practising correct posture and doing regular and deep inhales and exhales. These rhythmical movements done without resistance will gradually wind down your strength-training session. A cool-down will lead to a smooth transition from a higher-than-normal level of intensity to your usual degree of functioning.

Stretching

You should stretch your working muscles after each set and stretch your whole body after your cool-down. Stretching must be gentle and should be done so that you never strain your joints. You should especially avoid straining your back. Refer to p. 94 for basic stretching exercises.

In this chapter, I describe, step-by-step, the execution of some basic strength-training exercises. You can include them in your initial program according to your individual needs and abilities. If you start strength training after an extended period of sedentary life, choose only a few, less-difficult exercises. Add more and increase the level of difficulty as your strength gradually improves.

EXERCISES FOR THE LOWER BODY

Dumbbell Squat

Muscles participating:

Gluteals and quadriceps (prime movers); hamstrings, calves, spinal erectors, upper trapezoids, (secondary movers and postural stabilizers)

PREPARATIONS

- Hold dumbbells so that your palms are facing your thighs.
- Position your feet so that they are parallel and shoulder-width apart.
- Look straight ahead and adjust your posture so that your back is erect, your shoulders are back, and your weight is distributed evenly on both feet.
- Exhale fully.

Downward (negative) movement phase:

- Slowly lower into a squat as you inhale and maintain correct posture while keeping your legs parallel until you feel comfortable. You can stop at any point. Never descend any further than when your butt is level with your knees.

Upward (positive) movement phase:

- Start upward movement by slowly straightening your legs and exhale.

Common mistakes:

- Maintaining incorrect posture by drawing up your shoulders and not keeping your back straight
- Starting the downward movement phase by leaning forward and not by pushing your butt back and bending your knees
- Pushing the knees inward or outward so that they are out of parallel position
- Raising your heels

Easier versions of the squat are:

- Performing the movement without resistance (without the dumbbells), with hands on

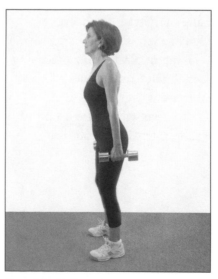

Dumbbell Squat

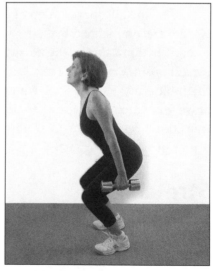

Dumbbell Squat

hips and elbows drawn back
- Standing up from a chair or bench with hands on hips and elbows drawn back
- Standing about a foot away from a wall with your butt and elbows against the wall when you squat

Heel Raises

Muscles participating:

Calves (prime movers), quadriceps, hamstrings (assisting)

PREPARATIONS

- Stand in front of a wall and place your palms on the wall at shoulder height and shoulder-width apart.
- Step back and fully extend your arms until you lean against the wall at a slight angle.
- Look straight ahead, raise your chest, draw in your abdomen, then inhale.

Upward (positive) movement phase:

- Start exhaling and slowly raise your heels until you are on the

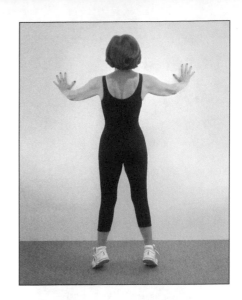

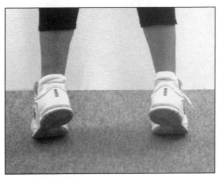

Heel Raises

balls of your feet. Hold the position for a moment.

Downward (negative) movement phase:

- Slowly lower your heels and inhale. (If you slightly bend your knees, there will be more muscle action from the soleus than from the gastrocnemius muscle.)

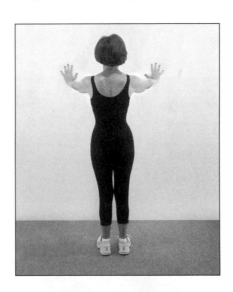

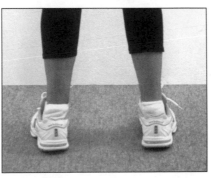

Heel Raises

Leg Abduction (Lateral Leg Raise)

Muscles participating:
Gluteus medius and minimus

PREPARATIONS

- Stand facing a wall and place your palms on the wall at shoulder height and slightly wider than shoulder width.
- Step back a little and extend your arms until you lean against the wall at a slight angle.
- Make sure that your weight is distributed evenly on both feet.
- Look straight ahead, raise your chest, draw in your abdomen, then inhale.

Upward (positive) movement phase:

- Raise one straightened leg laterally as you exhale. Raise it slowly and as high as you can without straining and hold for a moment.

Downward (negative) movement phase:

- Slowly lower your leg in a controlled manner as you inhale.

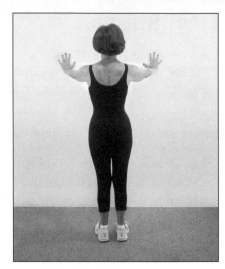

Leg Abduction

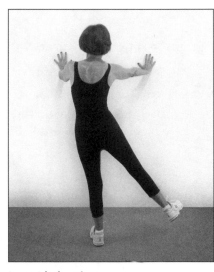

Leg Abduction

Forward Lunge

Muscles participating:
Quadriceps and gluteals (as primary movers), hamstrings and calves (as secondary movers)

PREPARATIONS

- Stand erect and look straight ahead with shoulders back and chest up. Your arms hang freely at your sides with palms facing your thighs.

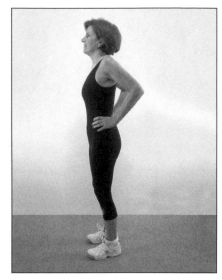

Forward Lunge

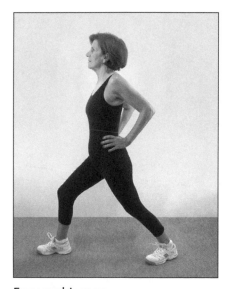

Forward Lunge

Forward (negative) movement phase:

- Lift one leg and lunge forward as you inhale. Make sure that you stay within your comfortable range of motion. Land on the full surface of your foot. At the end of the forward lunge, your knee should be above the toes of your foot. Pause for a moment.

Backward (positive) movement phase:

- Push back and exhale during this phase.

Leg Adduction

Muscles participating:
Adductor magnus, adductor brevis, adductor longus, and gracilis

PREPARATIONS

- Lie on the exercise mat with your knees flexed at 90°. Your feet should be flat on the floor somewhat wider than shoulder width. Place the exercise ball between your knees.

Inward (positive) movement phase:

- Inhale. Start exhaling and press the small of your back down into the exercise mat while slowly squeezing the exercise ball with your knees in a controlled manner. Hold the squeeze for a moment at the end of the motion.

Outward (negative) movement phase:

- Slowly release your knees' pressure on the ball as you inhale.

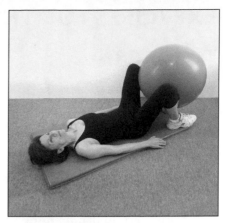

Leg Adduction

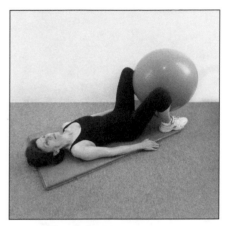

Leg Adduction

EXERCISES FOR THE TRUNK

Trunk Curls

Muscles participating:

Rectus abdominus

PREPARATIONS

- Lie on your back on a mat with your knees flexed at 110°–120°. Put your hands under the nape of your neck to maintain the neutral alignment of your neck. Inhale.

Upward (positive) movement phase:

- Press the small of your back into the mat while contracting your abs and slowly raising your shoulders. Hold for a moment. Exhale as you perform this upward movement.

Downward (negative movement):

- Slowly lower your shoulders

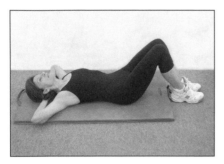

Trunk Curls

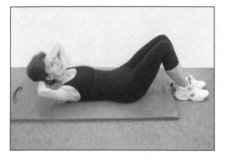

Trunk Curls

and inhale. **Caution:** Avoid using your hands to raise your neck. Trying to gain momentum by raising your neck with your hands will result in incorrect and less effective execution of the exercise and may also harm your neck.

Trunk Cross Curl with Knee Pull

Muscles participating:

Abdominal obliques, rectus abdominus

PREPARATIONS

- Lie on the mat on your back with your knees bent at 110°–120°. Put your hands under the nape of your neck to support the neutral alignment of your neck. Inhale.

Upward (positive) movement phase:

- Press the small of your back slowly into the mat while raising your left knee and right shoulder simultaneously. Rotate your trunk slowly so that your right elbow moves toward your left knee and, if you can, touch your left knee with your right elbow. Hold for a moment. Exhale during this upward movement. (After the downward movement, repeat the motion with your right knee and left shoulder, moving your left elbow toward your right knee.)

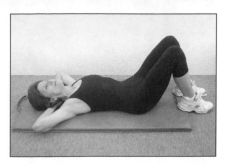

Trunk Cross Curl with Knee Pull

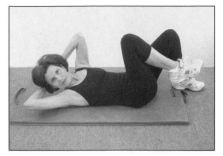

Trunk Cross Curl with Knee Pull

Downward (negative) movement phase:

*   Slowly and simultaneously lower your left knee and your right elbow back to the starting position. Inhale during the downward phase. **Caution:** Avoid using your arms to assist in rotating your trunk upwards. Your hands behind your neck should do no more than support the neutral alignment of your neck. Gaining any momentum by raising your neck with your hands will result in incorrect execution of the exercise and may also strain your neck.

Assisted Bent-Knee Trunk Curl

Muscles participating:
Rectus abdominus

PREPARATIONS

*   Lie on your back on a mat with your knees bent at 110°–120°. Your arms should be on the floor at your sides with the palms facing down. Inhale.

Upward (positive) movement phase:

*   Press the small of your back into the mat and contract your abs while pushing your elbows and forearms downward against the mat and slowly curling your trunk upward in a controlled manner. Exhale during this upward movement. Pause for a moment at the top of the motion.

Downward (negative) movement phase:

*   Slowly lower your trunk back onto the mat in a controlled manner. Inhale during this downward movement.

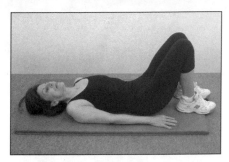

Assisted Bent-Knee Trunk Curl

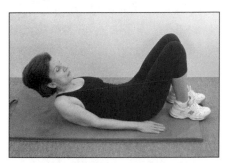

Assisted Bent-Knee Trunk Curl

Back Extension (Stability Ball)

Muscles participating:

Spinal erectors, quadratus lumborum, middle trapezoids

PREPARATIONS

- Place a stability ball under your trunk so that your chest, abdomen, and pelvis are fully supported by the ball. Hug the ball with your knees and arms. Your hands rest on the floor.

Upward (positive) movement):

- Press your pelvis and abdomen against the ball while slowly raising your elbows above your back as you arch your back, slowly extending it. Inhale during the upward movement. Hold this position with elbows drawn back and shoulder blades contracted.

Downward (negative) movement phase:

- Slowly lower your trunk back onto the ball in a controlled manner. Exhale during this downward movement.

Caution:

- This exercise must be done in a controlled and coordinated manner. Bouncing up or down on the ball will only compromise the effectiveness of the exercise and may strain your body as well.

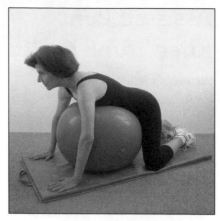

Back Extension (Stability Ball)

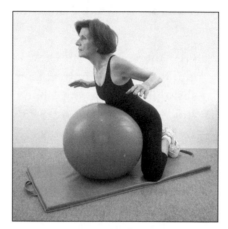

Back Extension (Stability Ball)

EXERCISES FOR THE UPPER BODY

Dumbbell Chest Press

Muscles participating:
Pectoralis major, anterior deltoids, triceps

PREPARATIONS

- Select two dumbbells of equal weight. Sit on one end of a flat bench so that your feet are shoulder width on the floor. Hold the dumbbells so that they are resting on your upper thighs.
- Slowly lower your back onto the bench while raising the

weights up to your chest so that they almost touch your chest. Your palms should face upward.

- In this position your legs are straddling the bench, your knees are bent at 90°, and your feet are flat on the floor. Inhale.

Upward (positive) movement phase:

- Raise both dumbbells in a slow and controlled manner until your arms are fully extended. Exhale during the upward movement. Make sure that you keep your head, shoulders, and buttocks in contact with the bench. Hold for a moment.

Downward (negative) movement phase:

- Slowly lower both dumbbells until they touch the sides of your chest. Inhale during this downward movement.
  Caution:
- Do not let your head hang off the bench.
- Do not arch your back when you raise the dumbbells.
- Do not bounce the dumbbells against your chest when you lower them and then use the momentum to raise them.
- If you feel any pain in your lower back, avoid straining the lumbar area by resting your feet on a stool in front of the bench. If you feel any pain in the shoulder area, stop the downward movement slightly before the chest.

One-Arm Rowing

Muscles participating:
Latissimus dorsi, biceps

PREPARATIONS

- Place a dumbbell on the floor along one side of the bench and stand behind the dumbbell. Place the knee that is closest to the bench on the bench. Keep the other leg straight and your foot flat on the floor. Lean forward and grip the end of the bench with one hand. With your other hand, reach down for the dumbbell and hold it so that

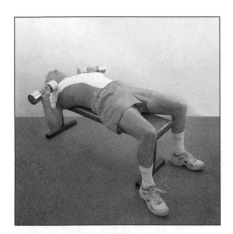

Dumbbell Chest Press

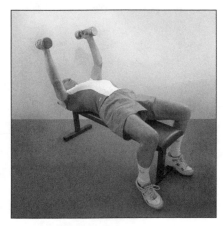

Dumbbell Chest Press

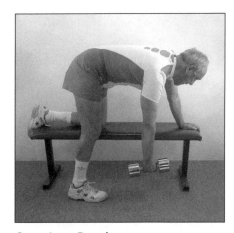

One-Arm Rowing

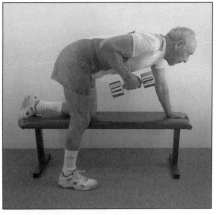

One-Arm Rowing

your back is straight and flat and your arms are fully extended.

Upward (positive) movement phase:

• Slowly raise the dumbbell toward your hip in a controlled manner. Hold the position at the end of the movement for a moment.

Downward (negative) movement phase:

• Slowly lower the dumbbell to the starting position.
• *Breathing:* One-arm rowing is one of those exercises when the (positive) effort is toward the center of the body. Many prefer to inhale through the upward movement because it makes the chest a more solid platform for the exercise. You may want to experiment with inhaling through the positive (upward) movement and exhaling during the negative (downward) movement and see which one you prefer. If you think this creates confusion, then stick with the general rule of exhaling during the positive (upward) movement.

Caution:
• Do not hunch or overextend your back.
• Place your knee on the bench right under your hip and keep the leg you stand on parallel with it to ensure that your back is not strained.
• Do not overextend the downward movement.

Dumbbell Chest Fly

Muscles participating:
Pectoralis major, anterior deltoid, biceps

PREPARATIONS

• Select two dumbbells of equal weight. Sit on one end of a flat bench so that your feet are shoulder width on the floor. Hold the dumbbells so that they rest on your upper thighs.
• Slowly lower your back on the bench while raising the weights up to your chest. Hold them about 12 in (30.5 cm) away from the sides of your shoulders at shoulder level with your palms facing each other. Your elbows should be bent a little less than 90°.
• In this position your legs are straddling the bench, your knees are bent at 90°, and your feet are flat on the floor. Your head, shoulders, and buttocks should be in contact with the bench. (Do not overextend your back.)
• Inhale.

Upward (positive) movement phase:

• Slowly raise the two dumbbells in a controlled manner until the dumbbells touch each other and your elbows stay bent slightly at the top of the movement.
• Exhale during the upward movement. Hold for a moment.

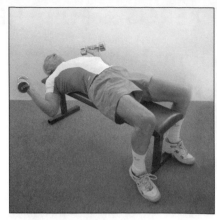

Dumbbell Chest Fly

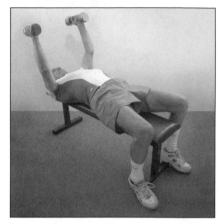

Dumbbell Chest Fly

Downward (negative) movement phase:

• Slowly pull the dumbbells away from each other in a slow and controlled manner and lower them while decreasing the angle at which your elbows are bent until they are bent a little less then 90° at the end of the motion when the dumbbells are level with the top of your chest.
• Inhale during the downward movement.

Caution:
• Do not let your head hang off the bench.
• Do not arch back when you raise the dumbbells.
• Make sure that your elbows are

slightly bent at the top of the movement and about 90° bent at the bottom. It is very important that your elbows never exceed 90° at the bottom of the movement. If you extend your elbows more than 90°, you may strain your shoulders.

- Always keep your wrists straight. Make sure that your hands are always in line with your forearms. It is a common mistake to put strain on the sensitive wrist joints by bending them.
- Never lower the dumbbells below the level of your chest and never raise them suddenly with a countermovement.
- If you feel strain in the chest or shoulder area, decrease the movement range so that the dumbbells are above the level of your chest at the bottom of the motion.
- If you feel pain in the lower back, rest your feet on a stool in front of the bench.

Chest Pullover

Muscles participating:

Latissimus dorsi, triceps

PREPARATIONS

- Select one dumbbell. Sit on the end of a bench with both hands holding the shaft of the dumbbell parallel with your torso, palms facing each other. Slowly lower yourself onto your back and raise the dumbbell above your chest. Put both thumbs under the shaft and cup both hands, one over the other, around one end of the dumbbell. Slowly lift the dumbbell with both hands and hold it with arms slightly flexed right above your head. Your head is positioned at the end of the bench, your back and buttocks are flat on the bench, your feet are flat on the floor, and your knees are bent at 90°.

Downward (negative) movement phase:

- With elbows kept parallel, slowly lower the dumbbell behind your head. Make sure that your back is not overextended. Inhale during the downward movement. Hold for a moment.

Upward (positive) movement phase:

- Press your lower back into the bench slightly while slowly lifting the dumbbell above your head. While lifting, keep extending your elbows until they are just slightly bent at the top of the motion right above your head. Keep the elbows

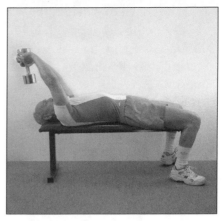

Chest Pullover

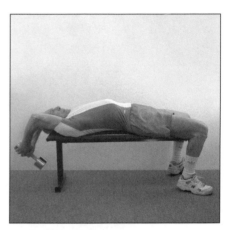

Chest Pullover

parallel. Exhale during the upward movement.

Caution:
- Always keep your elbows parallel and do not push them outward. Gradually decrease the angle of the elbows so that you start out with slightly flexed elbows and end up with elbows bent at 90° at the end of the motion behind your head.
- Lowering the dumbbell with elbows pushed outward or with straightened elbows will strain your shoulders.
- Do not let your head hang off the bench.
- Also make sure that (as with every exercise) you do not bounce back with a sudden countermovement, but bring

the dumbbell to a halt at the bottom of the movement, hold it for a moment, then slowly return it to the starting position.

• It is also a common mistake to arch your back while doing the chest pullover. This can strain your back. If you feel any pain in your back, put a stool under your feet.

Dumbbell Lateral Raise

Muscles participating:

Deltoids, upper trapezoids

PREPARATIONS

• Select a pair of dumbbells and stand with your feet shoulder-width apart and knees slightly flexed. Hold the dumbbells with arms slightly flexed so that your palms are facing your thighs. Make sure that your chest and chin are up. Do not push your head forward, hunch your back, or let your shoulders fall forward.

Upward (positive) movement phase:

• Slowly raise your arms sideways until the dumbbells are level with your shoulders and your arms are parallel with the floor. During the upward movement, keep your elbows slightly flexed.

• During this upward movement, keep your chest and chin up, and your shoulders and head aligned with your body and not slumped forward. Do not hunch as you lift the dumbbells. Your wrists must also be kept in neutral position—that is, they should be aligned with your forearms and not bent.

• Exhale during the upward movement.

Downward (negative) movement phase:

• Slowly lower the dumbbells in a controlled manner down to the starting position.

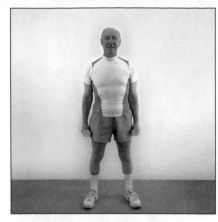

Dumbbell Lateral Raise

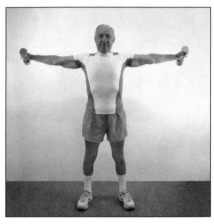

Dumbbell Lateral Raise

• Inhale during the downward movement.

Caution:

• Never attempt to lift the dumbbells above shoulder level. If you feel pain in the shoulders, you should stop the upward movement before the dumbbells are level with the shoulders.

• It is also a common mistake to let the dumbbells hang with your wrists bent. The hands always should be aligned straight with the forearms without being bent at the wrist in any direction.

Dumbbell Biceps Curl

Muscles participating:

biceps, brachialis, radio-brachialis

PREPARATIONS

- Select a pair of dumbbells and hold them with your arms at your sides and the palms facing the thighs. Stand with your feet hip-width apart and your knees slightly bent. Stand erect, with your chest and chin up and your shoulders level.

Upward (positive) movement phase:

- Slowly raise the dumbbells, rotating your wrists upward and keeping the elbows close to your sides and the upper arms aligned with your chest. When the dumbbells are at shoulder level, your palms are facing your shoulders.

Breathing:

- Biceps curls is another exercise in which the movement is performed in the direction of the body. Inhaling while raising the dumbbells expands the chest, which will provide a more solid platform for the exercise. You can try to inhale either during the positive (upward) or the negative (downward) movement phase and see which breathing pattern feels better. If this is confusing, stick to exhaling during the positive and inhaling during the negative movement phase.

Downward (positive) movement phase:

- Slowly lower the dumbbells simultaneously in a controlled manner.

Caution:

- Keep your back straight throughout the exercise. Do not lean backward or forward.
- Pause at the bottom of the motion for a moment and do not swing the dumbbells like a pendulum.
- Keep the elbows close to your sides and the upper arms aligned with the chest. Do not raise your elbows as you perform the upward movement.
- Wrists should always be aligned with the forearms in a neutral position and not bent.

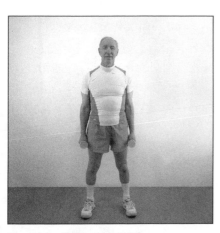

Dumbbell Biceps Curl

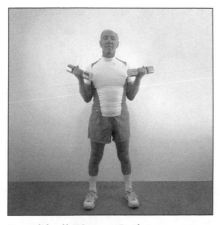

Dumbbell Biceps Curl

STRETCHES

BASIC STRETCHES

The function of stretches is to elongate and to relax our muscles and connective tissues, and to increase range of motion at our joints. There are some basic stretches that are safe and can be learned with relative ease. They can be applied after each exercise and/or after the completion of the exercise session.

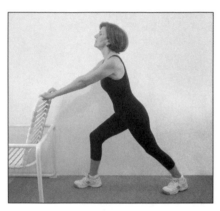

1. Achilles Stretch:

The Achilles Stretch elongates the Achilles tendon and the calf muscles. Do the Achilles Stretch after Heel Raises, Squats and Lunges. You should do this stretch after a long walk.

Executing of the Achilles Stretch:
Step forward and lean slightly against something like a wall, a table or the back of a chair. Slowly move your left leg forward, bend it and move your right leg back and keep it fully extended. Bend the front leg further and keep both heels firmly on the ground. Hold the stretch for about ten seconds and feel the stretch of the Achilles tendon and the calves. Switch legs and repeat.

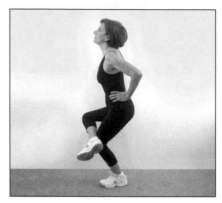

2. Piriformis Stretch:

The Piriformis Stretch elongates the piriformis and gluteus medius muscles. It also improves hip joint mobility. You should do this stretch after Leg Abductions and Squats.

Executing the Piriformis Stretch:
Stand by a wall and support yourself by leaning slightly against the wall. Bend your left leg and place your right leg right bent at about 90° right above the knee of your left leg. The ankle of the right leg should be slightly outside of the thigh of the left leg. Slowly lower your body by bending the left leg even more. Feel the stretch at the right side of your hip, buttock and thigh. To increase the stretch, push your buttock back slowly. Hold the stretch for about ten seconds. Repeat the same stretch by reversing the position of your legs.

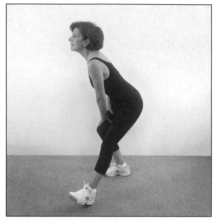

3. Hamstrings Stretch

The Hamstrings Stretch elongates the hamstring muscles on the back of your leg. It should be performed after Squats and Lunges and after a long walk.

Executing of the Hamstrings Stretch:
Step forward with your left leg and bend your right leg. With both hands above the knee of the right leg, bend forward a little. Fully extend your left leg and curl your toes back (dorsiflexion) so that only your heel touches the ground. Keep your back straight, Press your heel into the ground and push your buttock back. Feel the stretch in the back of your left leg and hold it for about ten seconds. Repeat the stretch with legs and position reversed.

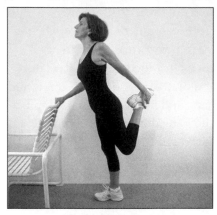

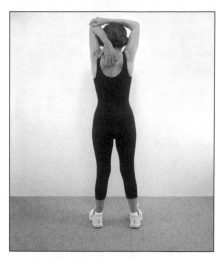

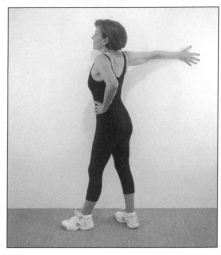

4. Quadriceps Stretch:
Elongates the quadriceps and ilionsoas (groin) muscles and improves hip mobility. Perform this stretch after Squats and Lunges and after a long walk.

Executing the Quadriceps Stretch: Support yourself by leaning against a wall, a table or the back of a chair. Lift your left foot by bending your knee and hold onto your foot with your left hand. Slowly start pulling your foot up and moving your left knee behind the fully extended right leg. Feel the stretch in the front of your left leg and in the groin. Hold the stretch for about ten seconds then reverse legs and position and repeat.

5. Triceps Stretch
Elongates the triceps muscles that run between the elbow and the shoulder in the back of the arm. Do the Triceps Stretch after Chest Press, Push-ups and after exercises that involve the extension of the arms against resistance.

Executing the Triceps Stretch: Lift your left arm above your head, bend it and lower your hand until the palm of your hand touches the base of your back. Lift your right arm and wrap your hands around the elbow of the left arm. Slowly pull the elbow in the direction of the center of your body. Feel the stretch between the elbow and the shoulder of the left arm. Hold it for about 10 seconds reverse your arms and repeat.

6. Pectoralis/Biceps Stretch:
Elongates the chest, anterior deltoid and biceps muscles. Improves range of motion at shoulder joint. Should be performed after Chest Flys, Biceps Curls and Push-ups.

Executing the Pectoralis/Biceps Stretch:
Stand with your right side parallel with and your right foot about 6 in. (15 cm) away from a wall. Step forward with your left leg and draw your right arm up behind your back until it is at shoulder height. Your right arm should be fully extended and the palm of your hand should be pressed against the wall. Slowly rotate your trunk to the left and feel the stretch in the right chest muscles, right shoulder and biceps. Hold it for about ten seconds, reverse position and repeat.

There are several more stretches that can be learned gradually as you progress with your exercise program. But these basic stretches will keep your muscles relaxed and you will experience a gradual improvement in your range of motion if you perform them in a regular manner after each exercise session.

Most fitness clubs usually have a wide variety of strength-training equipment. The range and complexity of this equipment may overwhelm someone not familiar with them. As a member, you are entitled to a demonstration of various fitness machines by qualified personnel. Take advantage of this opportunity and ask for an initial demo of the simple and basic machines. Make notes when you watch and listen, and do not hesitate to ask questions. Always be sure to learn how to adjust the machines for a perfect fit and how to load and unload them safely. It is better to become well acquainted with a few basic, easy-to-use machines for the legs, trunk, and upper body than to have a superficial knowledge of too many machines. A few weeks later you might want to extend your knowledge. Ask for another demo of the more complicated pieces of equipment.

When beginning a strength-training program, you do not need fancy, expensive, and complicated apparatus that takes up too much room, is difficult to move, and very hard to get rid of. Purchase only the basic equipment needed for your strength training. If, after comparing prices, terms and deliveries, and the cost of setup at several fitness stores, you buy a flat bench, a set of dumbbells, an exercise mat, and an exercise ball, you will have everything you need to start with. As you saw in the previous chapter describing various exercises, little equipment is needed for executing an effective strength-training program.

Although machines may be a safer bet to start with for a beginner, especially in a club environment where various distractions can lessen your attention and focus, free weights can be just as safe if you exercise carefully and effectively. If you decide to train at home, buy a flat bench, a starter set of dumbbells that are 5 lbs (2 kg), 8 lbs (3.5 kg), 10 lbs (4.5 kg), and 12 lbs (5.5 kg). You can always buy heavier weights later as your strength improves.

An exercise mat is also needed for certain trunk exercises and an exercise ball for core, balance, and functional training. There are various makes in various sizes on the market and depending on your size, the personnel at the fitness supply store will be able to recommend an exercise ball that is most suitable for you.

Beside equipment, you will also need exercise attire such as shirts, sweatshirts, pants, and a pair of shoes that are safe, do not obstruct movement, and wick away sweat. Make sure that the shoes fit snugly, that they do not catch on edges, that they provide ankle support and balance, and that they are appropriate for strength training. It is better to have cross-training or exercise shoes than running shoes because they provide better support.

Whether you are training in a club or at home, with machines and/or with free weights, it is very important that you observe and follow the rules of safety regarding exercise equipment and attire.

Visually and manually check that the equipment is safe and free of defects and is in good working order. Benches must sit firmly on the floor, plates must be secured properly on barbells and dumbbells (I have seen loose plates fall off and cause serious injury), and machines are correctly loaded and set.

Always remove equipment not needed from the area where you exercise. Always put unused dumbbells stacked on a rack. Even towels, your bottle of water, etc., should be placed out of the way so that you will not slip, trip, or fall over them.

Always make sure that no one in your close proximity is performing exercises, such as overhead lifts, that may lead to injuries if the person drops the weight, loses his or her balance, and falls.

Even seemingly little things, such as ensuring that your shoelaces are properly tied, may prevent an accident. Your clothes should fit well so that they will not hinder movements or get caught on equipment and cause a fall. Always have a towel to wipe the sweat off your face and hands.

You now have a sound understanding of what is involved in strength training and the method to achieve it, so it is time to carefully consider and weigh the pros and cons of training at home or in a fitness club, and hiring a personal trainer or exercising on your own. These are very important practical decisions that may influence the way you begin and continue with your strength-training program. It is worthwhile to invest some time and effort in considering these choices because they may affect both the process and the outcome.

Home Training or Training at a Fitness Club

If you live in a condo with exercise facilities, or a home with enough room to provide space for exercising, you might want to choose home training. Although you may not have the wide range and variety of exercise equipment that is available in fitness clubs, you may enjoy the convenience of not having to travel, park, change to exercise clothes, exercise, shower, change back to your regular clothes, and return home. On average, one spends more time on travel, etc., than on exercising unless the fitness club is within easy walking distance.

I train most of my clients in their homes. Even though the exercise area is often small and the equipment is sometimes only the basics, they get just as much out of each session as the clients I train in the best-equipped fitness clubs. Some of these clients let me set up their training facility and hire me to design a program and demonstrate the exercises, and then they continue their strength training on their own. When I visit them periodically to teach new exercises and plan further progression, they seem happy and satisfied with training at home. If you feel more comfortable at home and want the convenience of not having to join and travel to a fitness club, home training is certainly a viable choice.

On the other hand, if you are more comfortable in a fitness club and think that you will take advantage of the wide range and variety of exercise equipment and entertainment; if you enjoy the company of other members and want to try the various services (massage, fitness seminars, etc.) and classes (from yoga to pilates) offered at most clubs, then joining a fitness club is a sensible choice.

Before signing a membership agreement, you must make sure that you know everything you need to about the club, for example:

- Is the location convenient?
- How accessible is parking?
- What are the hours of operation?
- Take a tour at the time of the day when you will likely train and see if the place is pleasant or too crowded, too noisy with music blasting from speakers, etc.
- Check for cleanliness and orderliness of the exercise areas, locker rooms, and washrooms.

- See if the employees and members are polite, considerate, and courteous.
- Check the availability, variety, condition, and layout of training equipment.
- Ask about the rules of conduct.
- Ask about the qualifications of fitness personnel.

Generally you can ask for a one-month complimentary membership so you can try out the club's facilities before deciding whether or not to join. If a one-month complimentary membership is not available, ask for a few passes or just sign up for a month. Take advantage of this time and ask other members if they are happy with the services they receive. If you decide to join, take the agreement home, read the small print, ask questions, and if you are not satisfied with the clarity of the answers, you may want to further investigate certain issues. Clubs usually charge an initiation fee, want automatic bank withdrawals, and various other contractual commitments. You should sign only if you are completely satisfied with the terms.

Exercising on Your Own or With a Personal Trainer

Although most seniors are better off working with a personal trainer or fitness professional when they embark on a strength-training program, training on their own may be a viable choice.

If you cannot afford the services of a trainer on a continuous basis, you can always purchase a few sessions initially. This way you can at least have a starter program designed for you by the trainer. You should use those few sessions well and learn how to execute the exercises safely and effectively. If you cannot afford the expense of even a few sessions, you can buy strength-training books and videos and take advantage of the services of various community centers or learn from friends who are already exercising. This method could result in slower progress, and you may have to cope with the mistakes that go with learning to exercise by trial and error.

If, on the other hand, hiring a personal trainer in a club or at home is an option for you, there are certain important steps to be taken before hiring one.

Personal training is still largely an unregulated profession. There are trainers with excellent qualifications from internationally recognized institutions with very high standards, such as the National Strength and Conditioning Association (NSCA) and the American Council on Exercise (ACE). In these institutions, the education, theoretical, and practical knowledge of candidates is thoroughly tested and examined before they are granted certification and qualified to train others. Through a strict periodic recertification process (both the NSCA and ACE require personal trainers to recertify periodically), members of both are required to dedicate a lot of effort to keep their knowledge current and relevant through continuing education.

But there are a few trainers out there who obtained their certification via mail order from self-declared "institutions" or took a short course provided by a local community center and became "certified" by passing a low-level exam.

It is very important to make sure that the personal trainer you intend to hire is certified by either the NSCA or ACE or by an accredited college. Unqualified trainers may fail to help you achieve your goals or cause you harm.

Both the NSCA and ACE provide a referral service to personal trainers in your area (NSCA: www.nsca-lift.org or 1-800-815-6826 or 1-719-632-6722; ACE: www.acefitness.org or 1-800-825-3636 or 1-858-279-8227).

After making certain that the prospective personal trainer is well qualified and certified by ACE, NSCA, or has a diploma from an accredited college, I would highly recommend that you do some further checking to make sure that he or she has the necessary experience and disposition to train mature adults, e.g., qualities such as thoughtfulness, attentiveness, carefulness, dedication, and loyalty to clients, as well as compatibility, which are qualities beyond the ability of any organization certifying personal trainers to measure.

When you interview prospective personal trainers, it is important to ask for and check out referrals. You should also ask about their experience in working with seniors. You may also want to know what professional publications they read. This may range from bulletins issued by ACE and NSCA to the *Journal of Aging and Physical Activity* or the *Physician and Sports Medicine*. A more knowledgeable trainer improves the odds of you obtaining better results.

During the interview, you should pay attention to how thoroughly the prospective trainer interviews you about your medical history and condition, the medications you may be taking, and your fitness history and status. Does the trainer want your doctor's clearance and a fitness assessment? Ask for an initial program so you can determine whether the targets of that program are realistic and reasonable. Watch out for unrealistic promises—they are always a sign of carelessness.

I highly recommend that before any long-term commitment, you ask your prospective trainer for either a paid or a complimentary session in order to decide if the trainer demonstrates sufficient care and patience in teaching you how to perform the various exercises safely, correctly, and effectively, with proper breathing and posture; and if the trainer checks to make sure that the equipment and the immediate surroundings are safe and that training will take place in an injury-free environment.

You also want to know if the trainer has the personality and attitude necessary for motivating and encouraging you and helping you through periods of stagnation, inertia, and the occasional decline in your commitment to exercising. See if:

- the trainer is focused and disciplined and able to inspire focus and discipline in you
- he or she has a positive attitude that will motivate you to achieve your goals
- he or she has the energy, vitality, and inner drive to give the training process momentum, direction, and focus
- the trainer can recognize certain negative and positive factors in you and has the skills to influence and interact so that the positive factors prevail
- he or she can provide the necessary emotional support to keep you focused on achieving your goals

When I teach personal trainers, I find that most of them have the necessary knowledge to be good personal trainers, but only a few have the positive attitude and energy needed to inspire and motivate their clients. Few have effective psychological and interpersonal skills.

However hard it is to find such a trainer, the effort invested in searching for one will be paid back handsomely. Never resign yourself to a situation in which you are paying a trainer just to have someone to attend your sessions. Always ask, and sooner or later you will find a trainer who will be your guide and partner on your journey to a stronger and fitter body.

Case Studies

In this chapter, I will illustrate, through actual cases, how to commence and progress with a comprehensive and personalized strength-training program. I will also highlight the various problems—from mental blocks and obstacles to injuries—that some of my clients encountered.

Case #1

H. was sixty-five when she retired. She decided to live her life to the fullest. She came to the realization that everything she wanted to do— from playing the piano, travelling, gardening, and playing tennis—needed a strong fitness base.

She was healthy, with no restrictions or contraindication to exercising. At the same time, her state of fitness was below her potential.

Her physical assets were good flexibility; good coordination; and a well-proportioned body with healthy bones, joints, and muscles.

Her liabilities were some postural problems; a certain degree of muscle asymmetry; and insufficient lean muscle mass, which resulted in inferior strength.

Her psychological assets were an absolute commitment to play by the rules in order to improve her fitness, a great sense of discipline, and the ability to patiently persist until things worked out. As an additional bonus, she was eager to learn about her body, about good eating habits, about training in general, and about strength training in particular. In short, she was ready to apply the same positive attitude and persistence to her physical training that had made her very successful in her professional career.

We agreed that the most important goal was to improve her posture and dynamic muscle balance through strength training.

We began with three parallel programs. The first program was corrective and the exercises in it consisted mostly of stability ball exercises to strengthen her postural stabilizers. That is, due to weak scapular (shoulder blade) stabilizers, her shoulders fell forward, and weak spinal erectors resulted in an incorrect curvature/alignment of the spine. We started with specific exercises designed to improve these specific problems with her posture. Once the stronger core muscles began improving her posture, she progressed to a wider range of stability ball exercises that, besides correcting her posture, improved the overall strength of her trunk and functional skills such as balance and coordination.

The method we adopted with this exercise modality was to start with three or four essential exercises that she did under supervision until she perfected them. Once she perfected them, she continued doing those exercises on her own, and during our sessions we learned and added new ones to her routine until she had two comprehensive stability ball training routines consisting of twelve exercises each, which she did on alternate days.

The second program, which accompanied the stability ball training, was her daily walk at a brisk pace for about 30 to 45 minutes. It was not just simple fast walking—she also paid attention to correct posture, efficient gait, and correct breathing.

In tandem with the corrective program aimed at improving posture and muscle balance and the aerobic program to improve her cardiovascular fitness, we also started on a progressive strength-training program. Three times a week, we exercised with free weights to improve her general strength.

We were very cautious with the pace of progression. The emphasis was on improving quality, form, and technical correctness rather than on increasing the volume and intensity of the workouts. Exercises had to be performed with proper posture, proper breathing, proper coordination, and in their full range of motion.

We applied the following method to maintain progression:

- For each of the exercises that made up her initial program, we determined the ideal resistance. To be on the safe side, we chose a resistance against which she was able to perform each strength-training exercise eight times technically correctly and without straining. In order to give the body plenty of opportunity to learn and imprint the correct execution of each exercise, we determined the number of consecutive sets at three, with stretching between each set.

- As I have mentioned before, the focus was on perfecting technique. The exercises had to be performed slowly and in a controlled manner, and with fluid and coordinated movements in their full range of motion. We also made sure that she maintained both correct posture and breathing pattern throughout each exercise.

- Once all aspects of technique were perfected, we gradually increased the number of repetitions from eight to ten to 12 to 14, and then to 16 for each set.

- Once she could easily and correctly perform three sets of 16 repetitions of each exercise in this initial program, instead of the usual routine of increasing resistance by five percent, we learned new exercises instead. We did not want to fall into the trap of strengthening only certain muscle groups while neglecting others.

- Only after increasing the variety and complexity of strength-training exercises to a degree where every important muscle group in her body received regular and systematic training did we increase the resistance by five percent (and at the same time reduce the number of repetitions to eight per set).

Because she wanted to excel in tennis, we made sure that her trunk muscles were strong. It is the trunk in which forces find their platform to initiate motion, and enhance or cancel out each other. That is, the trunk must be strong because it must provide a solid platform for the various forces initiating different motions. It is very important that the muscles of the trunk are not only able to generate force, but are able to withstand the torque and the shearing forces of the sudden countermovements common in tennis. We added more exercises to improve the strength of the muscles in her midsection. We also progressed into complex, structural exercises that improved muscle strength not in isolation, but in the complex context of function.

H. maintained her interest in learning more and more about training, nutrition, and stress management. Thanks to her commitment, discipline, focus, and determination to improve her fitness, after four years of training, she managed to reduce her biological age by more than ten years. Her tennis improved to such a degree that she is able to play with and compete against younger players. Her improved strength and posture positively affected her piano playing. Now she does most of her training on her own and remains as committed and disciplined as ever.

I found that H.'s greatest strength was the absolute and unwavering commitment to improve her fitness.

Case #2

J. was about 50 lbs (23 kg) overweight and was very out of shape. Due to a combination of bad eating habits, inactivity, and excess weight, he had high blood pressure and a narrowing of the coronary arteries.

Before starting any serious training, he had to reduce his weight. Even his ability to walk for any extended period of time that could have been considered aerobic was compromised by the extra pounds he had to carry. His breathing was shallow, frequent, irregular, and inefficient because of the large deposit of subcutaneous fat in the stomach area.

After the initial assessment, it was obvious that he had to do more than gradually improve his eating habits. We agreed that the number one goal was reducing his weight. Until he consulted an excellent nutritionist, who refined the Spartan diet I immediately imposed on him, he ate fresh and steamed green vegetables and vegetable juices that were low in calories and very high in fiber. (To make the vegetable juices high in fiber, he added freshly ground flaxseed.) I told him to immediately eliminate saturated fat, trans-fats that might entirely close his already badly narrowed coronary arteries. He also had to eliminate simple carbohydrates and every carbohydrate that was above 30 in the glycemic index, as well as processed foods and red meat. He was supposed to eat very small portions six or seven times a day.

I told him to walk daily without straining himself. The establishment of an efficient but relaxed breathing pattern was the most important aspect of his cardiovascular training.

At the same time, we embarked on a comprehensive strength-training program. The idea was to combine a low-calorie, high-fiber diet; moderate aerobic exercise; and moderate strength training (which would build muscle, a metabolically very active tissue) that would reduce his weight and blood pressure and progressively improve his capacity to train more. We did strength training three times a week. He had a solid muscle base, but due to inactivity and overeating and the resulting obesity, his muscles were stiff and dysfunctional, able to produce only uncoordinated movements within a seriously restricted range of motion.

At the beginning, he had muscle soreness for weeks, even if we worked with relatively light weights. However, he persisted. His muscles responded well, and through a series of positive adaptations, they became stronger and functional. A few months later, J. started sea kayaking.

Due to the combination of dramatically improved eating habits, regular aerobic exercise and strength training (resulting in an active and functional musculature), and a new interest in a healthy and inspiring activity such as sea kayaking, he lost 30 lbs (14 kg) in six months. In a year his blood pressure was normal and consecutive medical examinations showed a gradual increase and improvement in the diameter of his coronary arteries.

After several tests confirmed his increased ability to train, we added snowshoeing to his winter aerobic exercise regimen. In his strength-training program, we focused on improving his muscle endurance by increasing the number of repetitions to 20 or more for each set.

He perfected his kayaking skills and improved his muscle endurance to such a degree that, after a year and a half of training, he could paddle at racing speed for 4.5 miles (7 km) as a member of a masters quadrathlon team. He also went on several kayaking trips to Northern Ontario lakes, where he was able to paddle for hours in rough water.

J.'s strength was his *ability to recognize that his lifestyle habits were leading to a disaster and to take immediate action.* His assets were his commitment to change, his persistence to continue with his exercise program, and his good lifestyle habits. This enabled him to achieve a lot more than he ever envisioned when he decided to lose a few pounds.

Case #3

M. and N. are a wonderful couple. M. was frail and, due to inactivity, her strength to function and perform movements were seriously compromised. The inactivity resulted in low functional abilities, muscle atrophy, and osteoporosis.

Her strengths were the ability to recognize that she had to make substantial and immediate changes in her sedentary lifestyle and a commitment to work patiently and consistently on her general goal of becoming more fit. She was eager to learn. She was very precise in documenting, recording, and monitoring her daily activities and her body's responses to training. This helped her to work out independently after a few initial sessions and we got together only periodically to assess her achievements, to widen the range of her exercise programs, and to plan further progression.

Initially, we designed and learned a stability ball exercise program that helped her improve her core strength and coordinative skills safely and comprehensively. Once she perfected her daily routine, we embarked on a weight-training program of various anti-gravitational, weight-bearing exercises to improve bone mass and bone mineral density.

M. enjoyed working toward her goals patiently and consistently. She enjoyed both the process and the achievement of her targets. Her progress was gradual and steady. Her bones, joints, and muscles became slowly, but noticeably, stronger and her functional abilities improved. M.'s dedication became an inspiration for her husband N., who also began to exercise.

N. was overweight, had high blood pressure, and his level of strength and aerobic fitness were far below his potential. His flexibility and posture were at a point where they seriously affected his ability to function.

Following his wife's example, he was just as persistent and consistent in his pursuit of improved fitness. In a year, he not only lost weight, but his blood pressure became normal and the dizziness and headaches he had experienced subsided. While a few years ago he could not even imagine it, he now walks to his office daily and climbs stairs. They mutually encourage and motivate one another. They both reduced their biological age by at least ten years and enjoy a quality of life they deserve.

It is interesting to mention that with the few husband-and-wife couples I have trained, both the recognition that inactivity (and the resulting lack of physical fitness) was the single most important obstacle to maintaining their quality of life as well as the decision to do something about it originated with the wives. Husbands followed their wives' example after seeing the results.

Case #4

R. had serious rheumatoid arthritis, high blood pressure, and was overweight. She had just recovered from cancer and from the deleterious effects of chemotherapy, extreme fatigue, overall weakness, and a compromised immune system. Her capacity to move and function properly was severely restricted. Add to this her poor posture, ineffective gait, and restricted range of motion and her prospects for a fit, health, active lifestyle were not encouraging.

R. also led a very demanding, stressful, but physically inactive lifestyle. Her ability to cope with stress was almost non-existent, and her attempts to manage stress were ineffective and counterproductive.

We started with a stability ball exercise program. Because of her high blood pressure, we avoided exercises that had to be performed in the prone position with the ball, which would have put pressure on her chest and abdomen.

In concert with the stability exercises, we started on a program of beginning strength-training exercises. R. worked out each day, alternating the stability ball program and the beginning strength-training program. She also walked daily at a comfortable pace for 25 to 30 minutes.

As her strength improved, we added increasingly complex exercises to her two programs. We also added various breathing exercises.

I explained to her that the effects of proper exercise are as much mental as they are physical— that when she exercises, she must focus on every aspect of correct form, correct breathing, and correct posture and shut out everything else. Focus is key. She should regard it as a form of natural therapy.

R.'s sense of discipline, perseverance, and keen attention to every detail of correct form paid off. Her improvements were spectacular. In less than six months her functional abilities, strength, range of motion, posture, and gait improved significantly. She lost 15 lbs (7 kg) and reduced her biological age by five years.

Case #5

B. was overweight, her strength and aerobic capacity were way below her potential, and she had problems with joint flexibility. She realized that her fitness had to be improved when she decided to climb a certain mountain. It was the highest mountain in the southern hemisphere. She knew that she did not have the strength or aerobic endurance to accomplish that. She had only about three months to get herself into shape.

She had good potential that was unrealized because of her bad lifestyle habits—her terrible eating habits were the worst in destroying her health and fitness.

I recognized that her enthusiasm for the pursuit of this goal was a strong asset that would motivate her to accept a very strict and demanding nutritional and exercise regimen. In order to achieve that particular goal, she could be persuaded to commit herself to play by the rules. I had the impression that she had neither the discipline nor the patience to persist and stay on course without being inspired by a dramatic and immediate goal.

I told her that she had to follow precisely every prescription in her exercise and nutritional regimen because in order to perform the task ahead of her, her training had to push the limits of her body's ability to adapt. That one step over the maximum amount of physical stress that her body is able to absorb and react to in a healthy manner means injury or burnout or both. This might not only put an end to her goal of climbing a mountain, but might also adversely affect her health.

We started immediately with strength training. We focused on anti-gravitational, weight-bearing exercises, such as squats, and we quickly progressed into cleans (complex structural exercise) because she had to be able to lift and carry 50 lbs (23 kg) of climbing and camping equipment at high altitude.

Her aerobic training consisted of fast walking on a treadmill and instead of going for higher speed, we increased the angle of the treadmill as her strength and endurance improved.

She also had to change her eating habits, which were some of the worst I have ever seen; her meals consisted of all kinds of simple, processed carbohydrates, chocolate, and ice cream. It was late in the afternoon when we had our first meeting. My expression as I listened to the list of "foods" she had been abusing her body with must have betrayed my shock because even before I had the opportunity to comment, she asked me when I wanted her to change her eating habits. I told her "starting as of tomorrow" she had to change everything. I gave her a list specifying what she could eat and how much.

Her less-than-perfect eating habits and total lack of discipline in resisting bad foods became the grounds for the first serious conflict among the many that followed. Because I told that she had to change her eating habits "as of tomorrow," she took advantage of the twelve hours at her disposal and ate about three boxes of chocolates (the rest of the Christmas chocolates) that were "lying around" at her home.

To cut the story short, she did an excellent job with her climbing expedition, although her group did not climb to the summit because of bad weather.

Her fitness and health improved dramatically. She then took up kayaking and within just three years after she began to train, her team of master athletes won two consecutive quadrathlon World Cup events, and she herself won several gold, silver and bronze medals at Canadian and U.S. masters championships.

It was B.'s motivation, drive, competitive spirit, and enthusiasm that helped her achieve the incredible improvements in the quality of her life. However, she still lacks the discipline, patience, and persistence needed to maintain and improve her health and fitness independently. Her example shows that even if you lack many of the qualities usually needed to achieve lasting positive changes, a reliance on one or two positive traits can overcome the disadvantage of many unfavorable and counterproductive attitudes.

Use these case studies to inspire you on your journey toward a strong and health body whatever your age and physical condition might be.

See your doctor, take a fitness test, use the knowledge you gained from reading this book, set your sights on a reasonable goal, and draw up an initial program that will lead you there. Do your first wall push-up and your first wall squat. Through increased strength, energy, and vitality, you will enjoy the rewards of your efforts in a few months.

The combination of inactivity, unhealthy eating habits, and the inability to cope with stress is the underlying cause of the physical decline that reduces our ability to enjoy life and to function independently as we get older. In fact, this combination of unhealthy habits is notorious for reducing the quality of life of every age group in our society. On the other hand, everyone knows, intellectual or theoretically at least, the benefits of a physically active life, healthy nutrition, and effective stress management techniques.

Unfortunately, realizing the disadvantage or the advantage of something does not necessarily guarantee that constructive change or action will happen. Recognizing and comprehending is one thing; applying such knowledge in a practically useful manner is quite another. Between recognition and action, there is a mental inertia that must be overcome.

I find that the inability to act *now*—which leads to endless postponements, putting off the day when we commit ourselves to a cause—is the number one reason for the lethargy and resignation that keep people from embarking on the journey that will lead to a better life. You have only one life to live. Why not make it the best and most enjoyable?

What are some of the most common excuses I hear when I talk to older adults who are sedentary, overweight, but still unwilling to make that first decisive step? What is my answer to those excuses?

Too Tired

The less active you are, the longer you continue your bad eating habits, and the longer you delay dealing effectively with your stress, the more tired you will feel. The physical fatigue you feel is the result of inefficient circulation, stiff joints, and atrophied muscles. Your body is deprived of wholesome, quality nutrients. Stress takes away the energy you need to act.

Give it a try. Take a walk and breathe. Do a few exercises. Eat healthy foods. If a doctor told you to take a little white pill for 30 days and you will feel better, would you do it? Well, try exercise for 30 days. You will have more energy and will feel better. Once you have experienced a better lifestyle, you will be encouraged to continue and enjoy further gains.

No Time

Examine the way you spend your days. Put your priorities in order. Eliminate the useless, the unproductive, and the nonsensical. You will be surprised at the amount of time freed up for training. The time you allot to exercising is your best investment. If you think that you cannot make time for exercise now, then be sure to make plenty of time for illnesses and hospitals later.

I've Gotten to the Point Where I Am Unable to Effect a Change

How do you know? You might be experiencing plateaus and burnouts because of an ill-designed program. There is a chance that you are not performing the exercises in the program technically correctly. You might also be doing too little or too much.

If properly trained, there is a potential for improvement in everyone. If you do not experience improvement and progression, see your doctor and consult a health and fitness professional. Let them show you how to effect change, how to draw on reserves that have never been properly utilized, to find abilities where you see none. The last thing to do is to resign yourself to the fact that something does not work out and blame yourself for something that has nothing to do with your ability to succeed.

I Tried, But I Didn't Have the Motivation to Go On

If you don't succeed at first, keep persisting in a different manner. There are many roads that lead to fitness. Find your own.

Whatever road you choose, first commit yourself to making a change. Sign a self-contract. Specify and visualize your goals. Develop a plan to achieve them. Record and document the process—every step of it. Notice and appreciate the accomplishments, even the small ones. Remember that change occurs slowly, degree by degree.

Always think in terms of success instead of fearing failure. Every step you walk is a successful step, and every set of exercise you complete is a building block leading to a better and potentially magnificent edifice.

Always visualize yourself as healthy, fit, and strong. With your sights set on that goal, your heart and lungs will work better and your muscles will have extra strength to move you forward in that direction.

Listen to "can-do" motivational tapes and speeches. Learn how to encourage yourself with positive self-talk.

Seek out the company of like-minded people. Consider joining groups involved in recreational activities. Go to your local community center, YMCA/YWCA, or fitness club and see what they have to offer.

Reward yourself for persisting and achieving your targets. Go on a special trip. Buy that fancy mountain bike, the best walking shoes, the most comfortable workout attire.

Don't wait for a moment. The more you postpone signing your self-contract and completing and recording on your exercise sheet the first set of exercises, the less likely you will be to begin after you put this book back on the bookshelf. Take that important first step now, and the second and third will follow naturally. Before you know it, you will be on your way to becoming the stronger and fitter person you have always wanted to be.

BEHAVIOR-Change Commitment Contract

1. I, _____, will begin my behavior-change program immediately and will incorporate the following into my daily routine.

2. I will pay attention to and try to recognize physical, behavioral, and mental/emotional signs of stress and be aware of them. I will record the common adverse reactions to stress, which may include everything from overeating to negative feelings.

3. I will try to identify the sources of stress and be aware of them.

4. I will steadily work on improving my personal skills to cope with stress that results in fear, impulsiveness, anxiety, anger, preoccupation, and other negative feelings by:

   a. working on building a positive mindset that includes changing perceptions, reactions, and being more reflective rather than reactive

   b. using breathing, relaxing, meditating, reading, listening to music, etc., to prevent and cope with stress

   c. constantly reviewing and appreciating the progress I am making and rewarding myself

   d. enlisting the services of a professional counselor if I need outside support to do all the above

_____   _____
DATE   SIGNATURE

Stress Management Strategies

1. I listen to what my body is telling me:
   a. tightness
   b. slumped posture
   c. shaky hands
   d. sweating and night sweating
   e. headaches
   f. dry mouth
   g. rapid and shallow breathing
   h. lack of energy
   i. strained face

2. I am aware of the following behavioral signals and their sources:

Signal	Identify Source
Talking to myself/arguing	_____
Overeating/rushed eating	_____
Swearing	_____
Outbursts of anger	_____
Nagging others	_____
Increase in bad habits	_____
Withdrawing	_____
Working more and making mistakes	_____

3. I am aware of the following emotional signs:

fear	_____
anger	_____
worrying	_____
loss of sense of humor	_____
irritation	_____

4. I employ the following strategies to manage my stress:
   a. Change my perception of things; acquire a sense of humor
   b. Reduce ambitions, lower expectations, become more realistic and accepting
   c. Learn to say no
   d. Get adequate sleep and rest
   e. Do breathing and various relaxation techniques
   f. Seek counsel

Behavioral Balance Sheet

Under the "Comments" columns, note when you feel each emotion.

Positive	Comments	Negative
Comments		
1. Sense of humor e.g., I laugh at myself		1. Fear
e.g., I feel fear when I have		
when I make a mistake.		
to go for a checkup.		
2. Calmness		2. Anxiety
3. Ability to reflect		3. Nervousness
4. Ability to say no		4. Outrage
5. Assertiveness		5. Indignation
6. Optimism		6. Preoccupation
7. Patience		7. Impatience
8. Discipline		8. Pessimism
9. Awareness		9. Annoyance
10. Ability to let go		10. Worrying

An Exercise/Lifestyle Commitment Contract

I, _____, pledge that:

• I will do strength training three times a week on the following non-consecutive days: _____, _____ and _____.

• I will adhere to the proper procedures of strength training, such as proper warm-up, correct execution of exercises, stretching, and cool-down, etc.

• I will walk briskly at least 30 minutes daily to improve and maintain my cardiovascular fitness and practise breathing exercises twice a day.

• In order to maximize my improvements and to fully realize my potential, I shall systematically improve my lifestyle habits, such as nutrition and stress management, practise breathing exercises twice a day, and give myself opportunities to relax. My short-term goals for the next three months are the following:

  a. Lose _____ lbs/kg.

  b. Be able to _____.

  c. Be able to _____.

• My long-term goals for the year are the following:

  a. Lose _____ lbs/kg.

  b. Lower my blood pressure to _____.

  c. Be able to _____.

  d. Be able to _____.

  e. Be able to _____.

• I will keep a daily record of my activities.

• I daily affirm my commitment to do all the above.

• I will find ways of rewarding myself for every improvement.

_____   _____

DATE   SIGNATURE

Program #   Lower Body/Torso

		Date:	Date:	Date:	Date:	Date:	Date:	Date:
Exercise:	RESIST:							
	1st set							
	2nd set							
	3rd set							
Exercise:	RESIST:							
	1st set							
	2nd set							
	3rd set							
Exercise:	RESIST:							
	1st set							
	2nd set							
	3rd set							
Exercise:	RESIST:							
	1st set							
	2nd set							
	3rd set							
Exercise:	RESIST:							
	1st set							
	2nd set							
	3rd set							
Exercise:	RESIST:							
	1st set							
	2nd set							
	3rd set							
Exercise:	RESIST:							
	1st set							
	2nd set							
	3rd set							

Program #   *Lower Body/Torso*

Exercise:		Date:	Date:	Date:	Date:	Date:	Date:	Date:
Exercise:	RESIST:							
	1st set							
	2nd set							
	3rd set							
Exercise:	RESIST:							
	1st set							
	2nd set							
	3rd set							
Exercise:	RESIST:							
	1st set							
	2nd set							
	3rd set							
Exercise:	RESIST:							
	1st set							
	2nd set							
	3rd set							
Exercise:	RESIST:							
	1st set							
	2nd set							
	3rd set							
Exercise:	RESIST:							
	1st set							
	2nd set							
	3rd set							
Exercise:	RESIST:							
	1st set							
	2nd set							
	3rd set							

Program #   Lower Body/Torso

		Date:	Date:	Date:	Date:	Date:	Date:	Date:
Exercise:	RESIST:							
	1st set							
	2nd set							
	3rd set							
Exercise:	RESIST:							
	1st set							
	2nd set							
	3rd set							
Exercise:	RESIST:							
	1st set							
	2nd set							
	3rd set							
Exercise:	RESIST:							
	1st set							
	2nd set							
	3rd set							
Exercise:	RESIST:							
	1st set							
	2nd set							
	3rd set							
Exercise:	RESIST:							
	1st set							
	2nd set							
	3rd set							
Exercise:	RESIST:							
	1st set							
	2nd set							
	3rd set							

Program #   Lower Body/Torso

Exercise:		Date:	Date:	Date:	Date:	Date:	Date:	Date:
Exercise:	RESIST:							
	1st set							
	2nd set							
	3rd set							
Exercise:	RESIST:							
	1st set							
	2nd set							
	3rd set							
Exercise:	RESIST:							
	1st set							
	2nd set							
	3rd set							
Exercise:	RESIST:							
	1st set							
	2nd set							
	3rd set							
Exercise:	RESIST:							
	1st set							
	2nd set							
	3rd set							
Exercise:	RESIST:							
	1st set							
	2nd set							
	3rd set							
Exercise:	RESIST:							
	1st set							
	2nd set							
	3rd set							

Program #   *Upper Body/Torso*

NB: Copy this sheet and file with your fitness documents

		Date:	Date:	Date:	Date:	Date:	Date:	Date:
Exercise:	RESIST:							
	1st set							
	2nd set							
	3rd set							
Exercise:	RESIST:							
	1st set							
	2nd set							
	3rd set							
Exercise:	RESIST:							
	1st set							
	2nd set							
	3rd set							
Exercise:	RESIST:							
	1st set							
	2nd set							
	3rd set							
Exercise:	RESIST:							
	1st set							
	2nd set							
	3rd set							
Exercise:	RESIST:							
	1st set							
	2nd set							
	3rd set							
Exercise:	RESIST:							
	1st set							
	2nd set							
	3rd set							

Program #   *Upper Body/Torso*

NB: Copy this sheet and file with your fitness documents

		Date:	Date:	Date:	Date:	Date:	Date:	Date:
Exercise:	RESIST:							
	1st set							
	2nd set							
	3rd set							
Exercise:	RESIST:							
	1st set							
	2nd set							
	3rd set							
Exercise:	RESIST:							
	1st set							
	2nd set							
	3rd set							
Exercise:	RESIST:							
	1st set							
	2nd set							
	3rd set							
Exercise:	RESIST:							
	1st set							
	2nd set							
	3rd set							
Exercise:	RESIST:							
	1st set							
	2nd set							
	3rd set							
Exercise:	RESIST:							
	1st set							
	2nd set							
	3rd set							

Program #   *Upper Body/Torso*

NB: Copy this sheet and file with your fitness documents

		Date:	Date:	Date:	Date:	Date:	Date:	Date:
Exercise:	RESIST:							
	1st set							
	2nd set							
	3rd set							
Exercise:	RESIST:							
	1st set							
	2nd set							
	3rd set							
Exercise:	RESIST:							
	1st set							
	2nd set							
	3rd set							
Exercise:	RESIST:							
	1st set							
	2nd set							
	3rd set							
Exercise:	RESIST:							
	1st set							
	2nd set							
	3rd set							
Exercise:	RESIST:							
	1st set							
	2nd set							
	3rd set							
Exercise:	RESIST:							
	1st set							
	2nd set							
	3rd set							

Program #   *Upper Body/Torso*

NB: Copy this sheet and file with your fitness documents

		Date:	Date:	Date:	Date:	Date:	Date:	Date:
Exercise:	RESIST:							
	1st set							
	2nd set							
	3rd set							
Exercise:	RESIST:							
	1st set							
	2nd set							
	3rd set							
Exercise:	RESIST:							
	1st set							
	2nd set							
	3rd set							
Exercise:	RESIST:							
	1st set							
	2nd set							
	3rd set							
Exercise:	RESIST:							
	1st set							
	2nd set							
	3rd set							
Exercise:	RESIST:							
	1st set							
	2nd set							
	3rd set							
Exercise:	RESIST:							
	1st set							
	2nd set							
	3rd set							

Program #   *Stability Ball Exercises*

NB: Copy this sheet and file with your fitness documents

Exercise:		Date:	Date:	Date:	Date:	Date:	Date:	Date:
Exercise:	RESIST:							
	1st set							
	2nd set							
	3rd set							
Exercise:	RESIST:							
	1st set							
	2nd set							
	3rd set							
Exercise:	RESIST:							
	1st set							
	2nd set							
	3rd set							
Exercise:	RESIST:							
	1st set							
	2nd set							
	3rd set							
Exercise:	RESIST:							
	1st set							
	2nd set							
	3rd set							
Exercise:	RESIST:							
	1st set							
	2nd set							
	3rd set							
Exercise:	RESIST:							
	1st set							
	2nd set							
	3rd set							

Program #   *Stability Ball Exercises*

NB: Copy this sheet and file with your fitness documents

Exercise:		Date:	Date:	Date:	Date:	Date:	Date:	Date:
Exercise:	RESIST:							
	1st set							
	2nd set							
	3rd set							
Exercise:	RESIST:							
	1st set							
	2nd set							
	3rd set							
Exercise:	RESIST:							
	1st set							
	2nd set							
	3rd set							
Exercise:	RESIST:							
	1st set							
	2nd set							
	3rd set							
Exercise:	RESIST:							
	1st set							
	2nd set							
	3rd set							
Exercise:	RESIST:							
	1st set							
	2nd set							
	3rd set							
Exercise:	RESIST:							
	1st set							
	2nd set							
	3rd set							

Program #   Stability Ball Exercises

NB: Copy this sheet and file with your fitness documents

		Date:	Date:	Date:	Date:	Date:	Date:	Date:
Exercise:	RESIST:							
	1st set							
	2nd set							
	3rd set							
Exercise:	RESIST:							
	1st set							
	2nd set							
	3rd set							
Exercise:	RESIST:							
	1st set							
	2nd set							
	3rd set							
Exercise:	RESIST:							
	1st set							
	2nd set							
	3rd set							
Exercise:	RESIST:							
	1st set							
	2nd set							
	3rd set							
Exercise:	RESIST:							
	1st set							
	2nd set							
	3rd set							
Exercise:	RESIST:							
	1st set							
	2nd set							
	3rd set							

Program #   Stability Ball Exercises

		Date:	Date:	Date:	Date:	Date:	Date:	Date:
Exercise:	RESIST:							
	1st set							
	2nd set							
	3rd set							
Exercise:	RESIST:							
	1st set							
	2nd set							
	3rd set							
Exercise:	RESIST:							
	1st set							
	2nd set							
	3rd set							
Exercise:	RESIST:							
	1st set							
	2nd set							
	3rd set							
Exercise:	RESIST:							
	1st set							
	2nd set							
	3rd set							
Exercise:	RESIST:							
	1st set							
	2nd set							
	3rd set							
Exercise:	RESIST:							
	1st set							
	2nd set							
	3rd set							